Research & Dissertation Writing for Postgraduate Medical Students

DISCLAIMER

The authors of the chapters in this book hold the primary responsibility for the contents of their respective chapters. The editors and publishers have accepted manuscripts in good faith and on the condition that all authors have adhered to the highest standards of publication ethics.

ISA
Indian Society of Anaesthesiologists
Eternal Vigilance

Research & Dissertation Writing for Postgraduate Medical Students

Editors

Madhuri S Kurdi
Professor
Department of Anaesthesiology
Karnataka Medical College and Research Institute
Hubli, Karnataka, India

Sukhminder Jit Singh Bajwa
Principal and Professor
Department of Anaesthesiology and Intensive Care
MM College of Medical Sciences and Research, Sadopur
Ambala, Haryana, India

Honorary Secretary
ISA National (2022–2025)

Academic Secretary
College of Indian Society of Anaesthesiologists (CISA)

JAYPEE

JAYPEE BROTHERS MEDICAL PUBLISHERS
The Health Sciences Publisher
New Delhi | London

JAYPEE **Jaypee Brothers Medical Publishers (P) Ltd**

Headquarters
EMCA House, 23/23-B
Ansari Road, Daryaganj
New Delhi 110 002, India
Landline: +91-11-23272143, +91-11-23272703
+91-11-23282021, +91-11-23245672
e-mail: jaypee@jaypeebrothers.com

Corporate Office
4838/24, Ansari Road, Daryaganj
New Delhi 110 002, India
Phone: +91-11-43574357
Fax: +91-11-43574314
e-mail: jaypee@jaypeebrothers.com

Overseas Office
JP Medical Ltd.
83, Victoria Street, London
SW1H 0HW (UK)
Phone: +44-20 3170 8910
e-mail: info@jpmedpub.com

EU GPSR Authorised Representative
Logos Europe, 9 rue Nicolas Poussin
17000, La Rochelle, France
Phone: +33 (0) 6 67 93 73 78
e-mail: contact@logoseurope.eu

Website: www.jaypeebrothers.com
Website: www.jaypeedigital.com

Inquiries for bulk sales may be solicited at: jaypee@jaypeebrothers.com

Research & Dissertation Writing for Postgraduate Medical Students

First Edition: **2026**

ISBN: 978-93-7202-629-0

Printed in India

DEDICATION

Dear postgraduate students and teachers,

This book is for you! We hope that it will make research and dissertation writing easy for you.

We dedicate this book to late Mr S Randhir Singh Bajwa (1944–2023), beloved father of Dr Sukhminder Jit Singh Bajwa, and to our families for always standing by us in the toughest of times, supporting us and encouraging us in our academic journey.

Madhuri S Kurdi
Sukhminder Jit Singh Bajwa

Contributors

Ankur Khandelwal
Associate Professor
Department of Anaesthesiology, Critical Care and Pain Medicine
All India Institute of Medical Sciences
Guwahati, Assam, India

Geeta Singariya
Senior Professor
Department of Anaesthesia
Dr SN Medical College
Jodhpur, Rajasthan, India

HG Manjunath
Director and Dean
Chamarajanagar Institute of Medical Sciences
Chamarajanagar, Karnataka, India

Former Professor and Head
Department of Anaesthesiology
Mysore Medical College and Research Institute
Mysore, Karnataka, India

Harsha Hegde
Scientist-F
ICMR-National Institute of Traditional Medicine
Belagavi, Karnataka, India

Jagadish G Sutagatti
Professor and Head
Department of Radiodiagnosis
Karnataka Medical College and Research Institute
Hubli, Karnataka, India

Laxmikant L
Professor and Head
Department of Community Medicine
Karnataka Medical College and Research Institute
Hubli, Karnataka, India

Madhuri S Kurdi
Professor
Department of Anaesthesiology
Karnataka Medical College and Research Institute
Hubli, Karnataka, India

Mahesh D Kurugodiyavar
Associate Professor
Department of Community Medicine
Karnataka Medical College and Research Institute
Hubli, Karnataka, India

Maneesha Godbole
Former Professor
Department of Community Medicine
Karnataka Medical College and Research Institute
Hubli, Karnataka, India

Manisha D Katikar
Associate Professor
Department of Anaesthesia
Ashwini Rural Medical College
Solapur, Maharashtra, India

Chief
Department of Neuroanaesthesia and Neurocritical Care
Balwant Institute of Neurosurgery and Intensive Trauma Care
Solapur, Maharashtra, India

Manoj Kumar
Associate Professor
Department of Anaesthesia
Anugrah Narayan Magadh Medical College and Hospital
Gaya, Bihar, India

Milon V Mitragotri
Assistant Professor
Department of Anaesthesiology
Karnataka Medical College and Research Institute
Hubli, Karnataka, India

Mukesh Kumar Prasad
Professor and Head
Department of Anaesthesia
Teerthanker Mahaveer Medical College
Moradabad, Uttar Pradesh, India

Nishant Sahay
Professor
Department of Anaesthesiology
All India Institute of Medical Sciences
Patna, Bihar, India

Parul Jindal
Professor
Department of Anaesthesia
Himalayan Institute of Medical Sciences, SRHU
Dehradun, Uttarakhand, India

Prasad S
Associate Professor
Department of Community Medicine
KAPV Government Medical College
Trichy, Tamil Nadu, India

Prashant Joshi
Assistant Professor
Department of Pathology
All India Institute of Medical Sciences
Mangalagiri, Andhra Pradesh, India

Prithpal Singh Matreja
Vice Principal
Professor and Head
Department of Pharmacology
Teerthanker Mahaveer Medical College
Moradabad, Uttar Pradesh, India

Ram S Kaulgud
Associate Professor
Department of General Medicine
Nodal Officer, Multidisciplinary Research Unit
Karnataka Medical College and Research Institute
Hubli, Karnataka, India

Ridhima Sharma
Associate Professor
Department of Anaesthesia and Critical Care
All India Institute of Medical Sciences
Nagpur, Maharashtra, India

Rohini Dattatri
Assistant Professor
Department of Trauma and Emergency
All India Institute of Medical Sciences
Mangalagiri, Andhra Pradesh, India

Sujatha MP
Professor
Department of Anaesthesiology
SDUMC
Kolar, Karnataka, India

Sukhminder Jit Singh Bajwa
Principal and Professor
Department of Anaesthesiology and Intensive Care
MM College of Medical Sciences
and Research, Sadopur
Ambala, Haryana, India

Honorary Secretary
ISA National (2022–2025)

Academic Secretary
College of Indian Society of Anaesthesiologists (CISA)

Ullasa Lingaraju
Senior Resident
Department of Anaesthesiology
Koppal Institute of Medical Sciences
Koppal, Karnataka, India

Foreword

ISA Indian Society of Anaesthesiologists

Eternal Vigilance

CISA

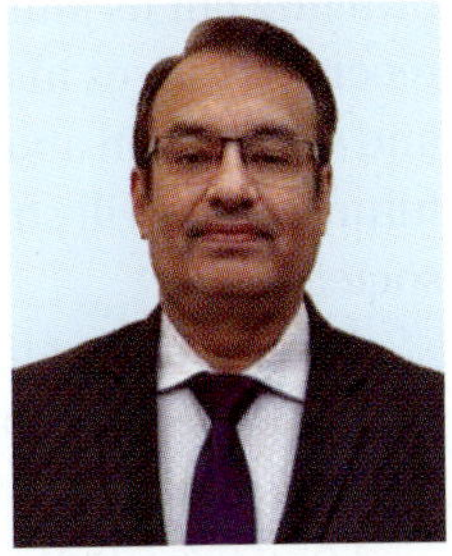

No medical stream can advance without research and academics. This is more pertinent, especially for anaesthesiology, which is a relatively younger branch, not more than two centuries old. For academic research to attain higher peaks, assistance is needed from several aspects, including administrative, financial, attitudinal, behavioural and, most important, from a knowledgeable mentor.

I have seen many an anxious student, researcher, and author running amok with a rejected thesis synopsis/dissertation/original article submitted to a scientific journal. At such times, the student or researcher blames the postgraduate guide or editor of the journal and vice versa. This means that the process of research and thesis preparation needs good knowledge of the basics of planning and conducting research and writing a dissertation. The student and the guide need somebody whom they can turn to for guidance at critical junctures. I am happy to say that this book "Research & Dissertation Writing for Postgraduate Medical Students" will do just that; it will serve as a very useful guide and friend to the students, teachers and researchers. It has chapters that focus on finding a research topic, selecting a proper study design, calculating the sample size, preparing a good synopsis, the ethics of research, how to confidently present the synopsis before the institutional ethics committee, basic statistics, presentation of the results, the examiners' analysis of a thesis and finally the various headings and annexures in a dissertation.

Obtaining the postgraduate guide's signature on the completed dissertation is often viewed as the victory point of the thesis writing process, and many a student has sighed in relief once the signature is obtained and the dissertation is submitted. However, in my opinion, this should not be the end-point. Every research should culminate in publication. A well-designed and conducted study culminates in its presentation at a conference and publication in a prestigious journal. This book gives tips on paper presentation and publication, too, which I am sure will bring smiles to the faces of the students and their teachers after the acceptance of their well-designed studies.

The book reflects the earnest effort of the editors and authors who as postgraduate teachers have literally lived the life of their students and have understood the problems and challenges of dissertation writing extremely well. There are plenty of textbooks on anaesthesia and other medical specialities but not many on dissertation writing, and I am proud to say that the College of Indian Society of Anaesthesiologists (CISA) has launched this book which will soon be a 'must-have' book for all newly joined postgraduate students and guides. This is the second book of the CISA; the first one was released at Chandigarh during the international conference ISA World SIVA Congress 2025. It is indeed a very satisfying moment for me when a book on research and publications is being published by the CISA; all the three domains, namely research, publications and ISA, are very close to my heart. Nevertheless, our esteemed society, the ISA mainly focuses on patient safety, anaesthesia education, and the enhancement of research activities.

It has been a satisfying career for me, having got an opportunity to work for ISA in various capacities, first as a National Governing Council member of ISA, then as Associate Editor-in-Chief of the Indian Journal of Anaesthesia and now as Hon. Secretary of ISA. The 3 years of working as Secretary of our prestigious body have been simply wonderful and fulfilling for me as I got the opportunity to help in establishing the CISA in 2023 and later on in coming out with its various academic projects, including bringing out its journal Practical Evidence in Anaesthesia Knowledge (PEAK), this book and books on recent advances in various streams of our subject. In fact, it gives me the feelings of self-actualisation and satisfaction about having done justice to our speciality; nonetheless, my efforts will continue in the future, and I will strive to live up to the expectations of more than 50,000 members of our prestigious society.

I am confident that this book will be recommended in the postgraduate medical curriculum by the National Medical Commission in the days to come and will shine on the bookshelves of all postgraduate medical students.

Long live CISA!

Long live ISA!

Jai Hind!

Sukhminder Jit Singh Bajwa
Principal and Professor
Department of Anaesthesiology and Intensive Care
MM College of Medical Sciences and Research, Sadopur
Ambala, Haryana, India

Honorary Secretary, ISA National (2022–2025)
Academic Secretary, College of Indian Society of Anaesthesiologists (CISA)

Message by the Chancellor, College of the Indian Society of Anaesthesiologists

Greetings from Dr J Balavenkatasubramanian!

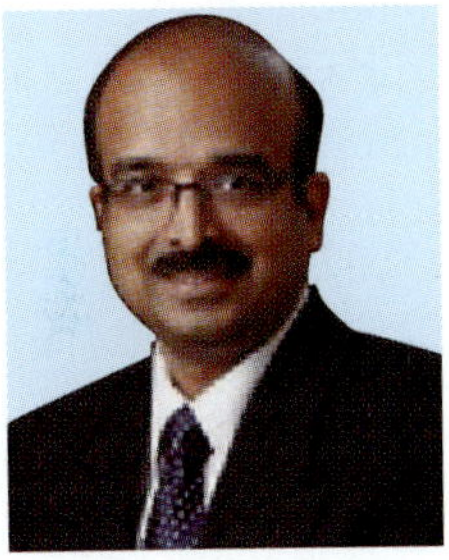

The nuclear thought of the Indian Society of Anaesthesiologists (ISA) in establishing the College of ISA (CISA) is to promote research activities in our country.

The best way to make this percolate is to reach the young residents as they pursue their education in the anaesthesia speciality.

I am so delighted to know about this book which I am sure would be a treasure for every postgraduate student and young anaesthesiologist who is about to embark on the journey of lucidly understanding the various facets of writing a dissertation, CTRI registration, ethical committee clearance, basic statistics, data collection, copyright issues, plagiarism and academic integrity.

This book would be a one-stop solution to every anaesthesiologist embarking on the journey of research and publication.

I congratulate and thank all the contributors with a special note of thanks to the authors for their hard work and effort in making this book a possibility.

Let this book inspire several anaesthesiologists to contribute to the literature.

In gratitude,

J Balavenkatasubramanian
President, ISA National (2024–2025)
Chancellor, College of ISA
Secretary, World Federation of Society of Anaesthesiologists (2024–2026)

Message by the Vice-Chancellor, College of the Indian Society of Anaesthesiologists

ISA Indian Society of Anaesthesiologists

CISA College of Indian Society of Anaesthesiologists

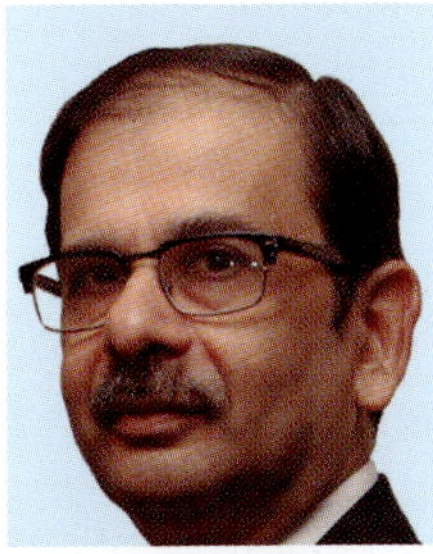

I am delighted to write this message for this book titled “Research and Dissertation Writing for Postgraduate Medical Students”. It gives me even greater pleasure as it is the second book to be launched under the aegis of the College of the Indian Society of Anaesthesiologists (CISA). The CISA was formally launched on 15 October 2024, and this is a landmark event in the history of the Indian Society of Anaesthesiologists (ISA). The CISA was formed to co-ordinate all the academic activities of the ISA. After approval from the Annual General Body Meeting at Gurugram, the structure and functional details of the CISA were defined, as was the tight bond with the ISA, the parent body, over the next year. The current structure of the CISA was approved by the Annual General Body Meeting at Patna in November 2024.

Writing a dissertation is an essential component of the postgraduate curriculum in almost all speciality and superspeciality subjects. The aim is to introduce students to clinical research methodology and scientific writing. However, there is often inadequate guidance available to students, and there is wide variability both in the quality of research and publication. There is therefore a crying need for a simple and practical yet elaborate and thorough resource to help students as well as teachers to navigate through research projects. This book “Research and Dissertation Writing for Postgraduate Medical Students” will fill this void. It has 15 chapters that take the reader through the journey from research idea to study design, protocol submission, ethical and regulatory issues, presentation and statistical analysis of data and writing the dissertation. Eleven appendices provide useful templates for various research tasks and submissions, and end with a useful FAQ regarding dissertation.

The chapters are written by experienced teachers and researchers. The book gets its stamp of authority with the eminence of its editors, Dr Madhuri S Kurdi and Dr Sukhminder Jit Singh Bajwa. Dr Madhuri S Kurdi is a renowned medical teacher and is the Editor-in-Chief elect of the Indian Journal of Anaesthesia. Dr Bajwa is currently the Secretary of ISA National. He has a strong inclination to academics and has extensive experience in publishing, both as an author and as an editor. He is the Editor-in-Chief of Practical Evidence in Anaesthesia Knowledge (PEAK), the official journal of the CISA.

I am certain that 'Research and Dissertation Writing for Postgraduate Medical Students' will become a beacon of light for the students and faculty of anaesthesiology in India. It has been my proud privilege to have been associated with the initiation of CISA (as President-Elect) and this book (as Immediate Past-President and Academic Chair). These are exciting times for the ISA and the CISA. I wish the editors, authors and readers of this book as well as CISA all the very best.

Jigeeshu V Divatia
Immediate Past-President and Academic Chair, ISA (2024–2025)
Vice-Chancellor, College of the Indian Society of Anaesthesiologists

Message by the Pro Chancellor, College of Indian Society of Anaesthesiologists

Dear Post-graduate Students and Teachers,

Namaskar!

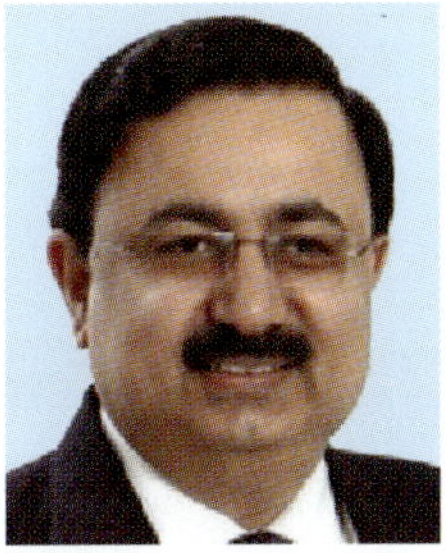

It is indeed a proud moment for me to write this message for the second book being published by the College of the Indian Society of Anaesthesiologists (CISA). This book on Research and Dissertation writing has chapters written by authors who are well experienced in their respective domains. The chapters are based on topics that include the various milestones of doing research and writing a dissertation, starting from deciding the topic of the dissertation, planning the study, writing the synopsis, presenting it before the ethics committee and then practically implementing the study followed by writing the dissertation. Nevertheless, I have observed in my journey of postgraduate teaching that not all students are good in scientific writing and most are naive about basic research when they join post-graduation. I am certain that this book will quieten the anxious minds of these fresher post-graduate students and will put to ease the post-graduate guides as well. It will also be useful to the clinical practitioner newly embarking on research.

I heartily congratulate the editors of this book, Dr Madhuri S Kurdi, an experienced post-graduate teacher in anaesthesiology; Dr Sukhminder Jit Singh Bajwa, well known for his passion for research and scientific writing and the authors for bringing out this book in a form which conveys simple and practical information on research and dissertation writing.

I wish this book the brightest success.

Long Live ISA!

Long Live CISA!

Naveen Malhotra

President Elect, ISA National (2024–2025)

Pro Chancellor CISA

Message by the Pro Chancellor, College of Indian Society of Anaesthesiologists

Message by the Dean
(Publication of Textbooks, Monographs, etc.), CISA

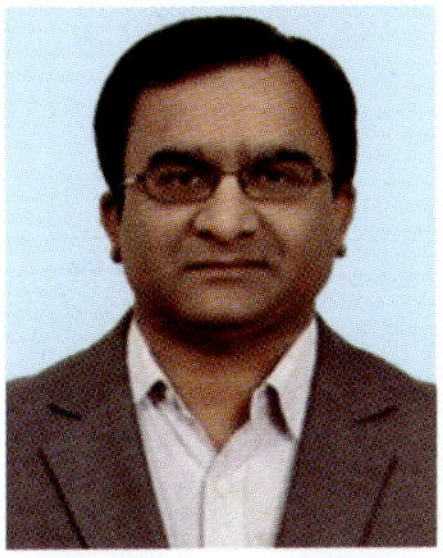

I am very much delighted to write my message for this book "Research and Dissertation Writing for Postgraduate Medical Students". This is the second book under the Deanery of Textbooks and Monograms of the College of Indian Society of Anaesthesiologists.

This book is unique and a need of the hour for all the postgraduate students in helping and guiding their dissertation work. Each chapter is written by faculty who have vast experience in dealing with post-graduate dissertation work.

The book gives excellent guidance on topics like research study design, ethical issues, clinical trial registration, plagiarism, data collection and statistics. I am sure that postgraduate students will benefit from this book and will be able to publish research papers and their dissertation.

My sincere thanks go to all the authors and editors for their scholarly work and immense academic contribution.

Rama Krishna Reddy Mudiganti
Dean, College of Indian Society of Anaesthesiologists (T&M Deanery)
Governing Council Member, ISA National
Professor and Medical Superintendent
Patnam Mahender Reddy Institute of Medical Sciences (PMRIMS)
Hyderabad, Telangana, India

Preface

Several years ago, we wrote our dissertations as novice scientific writers under the supervision of our postgraduate guides. We still remember those moments of ecstasy when we were allotted our guides, the moments of worry when we were choosing and groping for a good topic in the institution library and the moments of frustration when our guides were not happy with the topics that we had selected. Who can forget those moments of agony when we were bombarded with queries by the institutional ethics committee and were dangerously close to getting our synopsis rejected, those moments of hurry and impatience whilst getting the dissertation typed and bounded and our sighs of relief when our guides signed the final copy of the dissertation? From those moments onwards to the times in our journey of teaching and guiding postgraduate students, we have one common observation, that most postgraduate students embarking on a dissertation are ignorant and naive as far as research is concerned.

The newly joined postgraduate students are not aware of the basics of research, are not very good at doing a scientific search of topics for research and are technically inept at typing and formatting. Newly appointed postgraduate guides often fumble in finding a suitable topic of research for their students and senior postgraduate guides struggle with insincere students. As examiners, we often come across poorly written synopses, badly planned and conducted research studies and carelessly written dissertations. All these reflect poor effort by the teacher and/or student and teacher–student asynchrony. All of these motivated us to bring out this book.

This book has chapters written by well-experienced authors and postgraduate teachers on topics related to the preparation of a dissertation, namely the basics of designing a research study, calculating the sample size, preparation of the synopsis and its presentation before the ethics committee, collection and presentation of data, basic statistical tests for the observations and finally writing the dissertation under various subheadings. The culmination of the research as a paper/poster presentation in a conference or publication in a scientific journal is also discussed.

We sincerely hope that this book will be of help to all postgraduate students and guides and will enhance the output of good-quality research and publications from our nation. We are grateful to all the authors of this book for their hard work, dedication and commitment in contributing to the chapters. We are grateful to our postgraduate guides and teachers who have been inspiration and role models for us.

Finally, we would like to quote Lord Krishna, "*Karmanye Vadhikaraste, Ma Phaleshu Kadachana*". A good dissertation is sure to come up when the teacher and student do their work with sincerity and enthusiasm. As teachers, we should guide our students sincerely and without any expectations. We should accept the student as they are and believe in them because every student is unique. In turn, postgraduate students should respect their guides and take their valuable advice and blessings. A teacher's blessings and a student's gratitude are the oars that keep the boat of life rowing for both the teacher and the student.

Madhuri S Kurdi
Sukhminder Jit Singh Bajwa

Preface

Acknowledgements

We are deeply grateful to all our teachers, guides and students who have been a part of our academic journey.

Dr Madhuri S Kurdi
Dr Sukhminder Jit Singh Bajwa
Editors

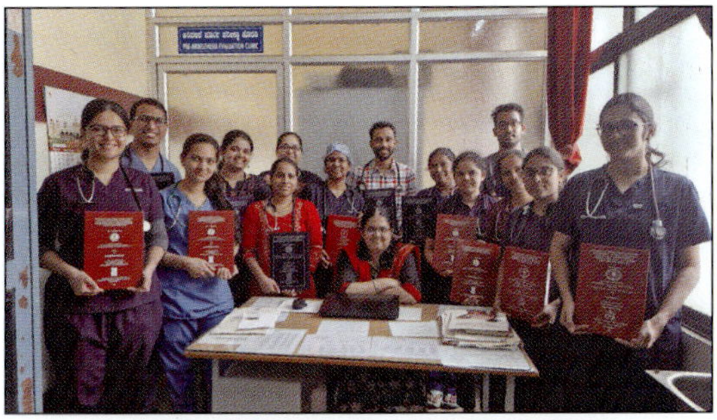

With my Postgraduate Students
—Dr Madhuri S Kurdi

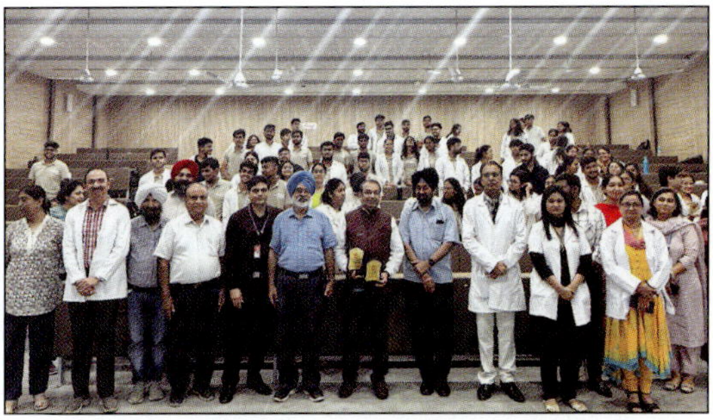

With my Medical Students
—Dr Sukhminder Jit Singh Bajwa

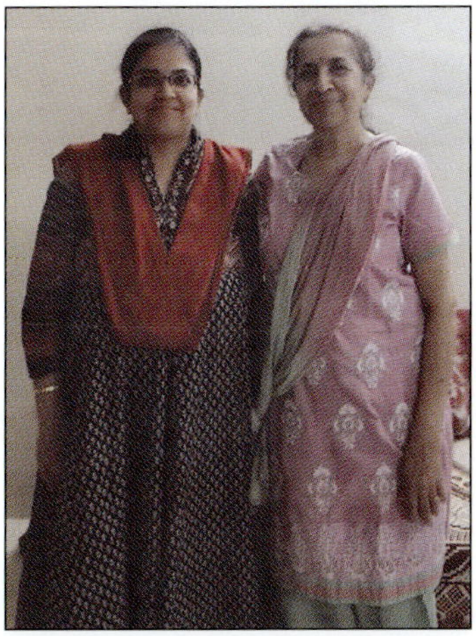

With my Postgraduate Guide, Dr Nalini Damle
—Dr Madhuri S Kurdi

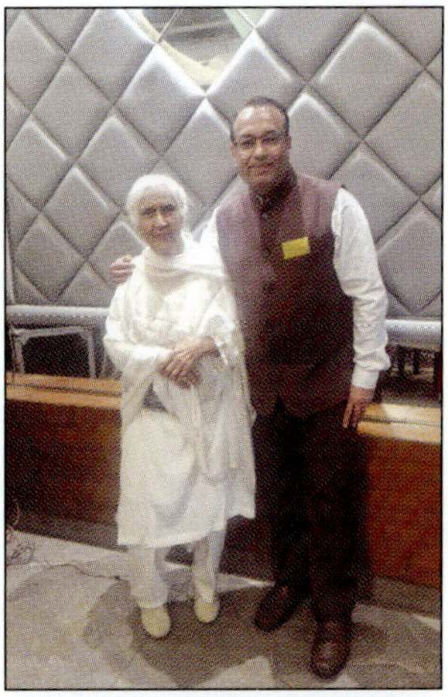

With my Postgraduate Guide, Dr Jasbir Kaur
—Dr Sukhminder Jit Singh Bajwa

Contents

Abbreviations of Units of Measurement

cm	:	centimetre
IU	:	international units
k cal	:	kilocalorie
kg	:	kilogram
L	:	litre
min	:	minute
mL	:	millilitre
mm Hg	:	millimetres of mercury
sq.m	:	square metre

1

CHAPTER

Introduction to Dissertation, Research, and Its Role in Medical Education

Madhuri S Kurdi

INTRODUCTION

Dissertation writing is an important part of the postgraduate (PG) medical curriculum. Every postgraduate student has to go through the process of dissertation writing. However, most students are naive and totally ignorant about the procedure of dissertation writing. This chapter touches upon the basic steps of dissertation writing and the qualities of a good research study.

STATUS OF RESEARCH IN THE MEDICAL CURRICULUM

Research in the undergraduate medical curriculum in our country is sparse and includes conducting Indian Council of Medical Research (ICMR) research projects and community medicine research projects. However, research has been given due importance in the competency-based medical education (CBME) postgraduate and superspeciality curriculum. The National Medical Commission and the National Board of Examinations mandate to provide teaching in research during postgraduation for Doctor of Medicine (MD) in anaesthesia and Diplomate of National Board (DNB) in anaesthesia, respectively.[1] Accordingly, a student is expected to carry out work on an assigned research project under the guidance of a PG teacher (guide appointed by the university) who will be allotted to the student by the Principal and Head of the Department soon after joining the course.

WHAT IS A DISSERTATION?

The results of the work that is conducted as a part of the research project are written up and submitted in the form of a thesis (dissertation). A dissertation is a practical exercise that educates students about the basics of research methodology, promotes scientific writing, encourages critical thinking, and inculcates an aptitude for research. The terms "dissertation" and "thesis" are often used interchangeably with the user not knowing their exact meaning. Nevertheless, both are scholarly pieces of writing based on research projects undertaken by students to complete a master's degree or PhD degree; however, the main difference is that a thesis is based on existing research and expands it, whereas in a dissertation, the student conducts his/her own research and then performs an analysis.[1,2]

STEPS OF DISSERTATION RESEARCH AND WRITING

The dissertation topic is allotted to the student by the PG guide in the first 3 months after joining the course. The topic is based on a research question. This process of formulating a research question can be challenging for both the student and teacher. The research question has to be Feasible in the student's clinical setup, Interesting, Novel, Ethical and Relevant (FINER).[3] The research question can be obtained from scientific literature research including articles recently published in reputed journals or from clinical observations in routine clinical practice.[4] Once the topic or research question has been finalised, the student has to plan the study design and calculate the appropriate sample size for the study after discussing with the statistician. The student will then prepare the synopsis and present it first before an audience including the department faculty for critical comments and later to the institutional ethics committee for approval. Once the ethics committee approval is obtained, the certificate of approval is attached to the synopsis. The synopsis is submitted online to the university by the college. It is examined by the examiners and either accepted or rejected. Review comments are sent online to the student and the student has to make corrections, revise the synopsis, and resubmit to the university for approval. Next, the student has to apply online for Clinical Trials Registry India (CTRI) approval of the study. Once the CTRI approval is obtained, the recruitment of the study subjects starts. The study cases are conducted during the study period (usually 1–1.5 years) and the student collects the concerned data and parameters and enters them in a study proforma and a master chart. The review of the dissertation work takes place at regular intervals in the department by the PG guide and the head of the department.[1]

At the end of the study period, the student has to apply statistical tests, taking the help of the postgraduate guide and a statistician in case the statistics are complicated. A conclusion is derived from the observations. The results are presented in the thesis in the form of appropriate tables and figures. The completed dissertation has to be written under several headings: Abstract, Introduction, Aims and Objectives of the Study, Review of Literature, Materials and Methods, Observations and Results, Discussion including Limitations of the Study, Conclusions, Bibliography, Summary.[1,5]

The list of annexures in the dissertation should also include the following:

- Proforma used for the data collection
- Informed consent form both in English and local vernacular language
- Master chart
- Institutional review board certificate
- Plagiarism certificate
- Certificate from Institutional ethical committee

Examples of the same are given in the annexure section of this book **(Annexures 1 to 5)**.

Other pages in the dissertation include Table of Contents, Certificate from PG Guide, Co-guide, Head of Department, Principal, Acknowledgement page and list of Abbreviations. The dissertation is presented online or in the form of bonded print copies, depending on the university rules and submitted to the university, postgraduate guide, and the department library.[1]

FLOW DIAGRAM OF DISSERTATION WORK

This flowchart outlines the step-by-step process of postgraduate thesis work—from research training and ethics approval to data analysis, thesis submission, and publication **(Flowchart 1)**.

The thesis is usually submitted at least 3–6 months before the theory and clinical/practical examination. It is examined by external and internal examiners of the university. The postgraduate student is allowed to appear for the theory and practical/clinical examination only after acceptance of the thesis by the examiners. In case of DNB students, the results of practical examination are declared only after acceptance of the thesis, though the student may be permitted to appear for practical examinations after submission of the thesis.[1]

Flowchart 1: Steps in postgraduate thesis work and research process.

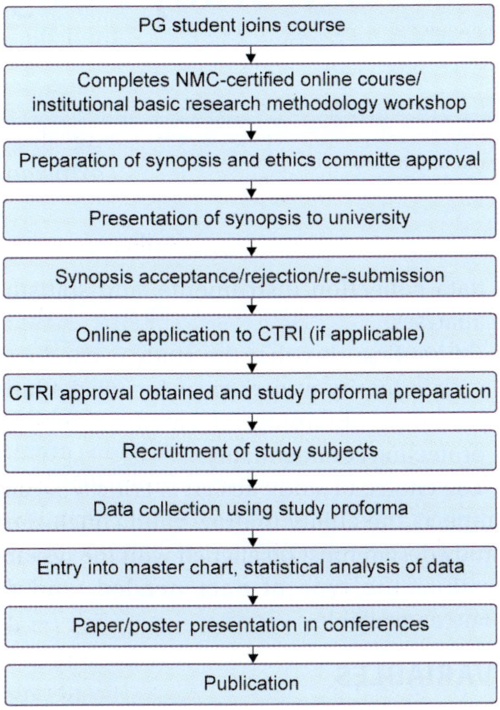

(CTRI: Clinical Trials Registry India; NMC: National Medical Commission; PG: postgraduate)

QUALITIES OF A GOOD RESEARCH STUDY[1,3,5,6]

- Research study designs and statistical tests can be of various types and they should suit the study topic and research question. Hence, it is important that the student doing a dissertation should have a basic knowledge of research study designs and statistical tests.
- Sample size calculation is done at the time of preparing the synopsis, preferably after consulting a statistician.
- The study population, inclusion/exclusion criteria, and study period are clearly defined.
- The sampling technique, method of randomisation, blinding, allocation, and concealment are clearly defined.
- The statistician who helped decide sample size also advises the appropriate application of statistical tests on study completion.
- The research is properly interpreted and observations are well presented in the form of appropriate figures and tables.
- The research question is novel and the results of the thesis can make a difference to clinical practice.
- The study is finally accepted for presentation at conferences including award sessions and in reputed journals for publication.
- The PG student develops interest in the topic of the thesis and acquires expertise in this later on in his career.

CONCLUSION

A dissertation forms a vital component of PG medical education. A good dissertation reflects the work of a seasoned, dedicated PG guide, and a sincere meticulous PG student.

REFERENCES

1. Harsoor SS, Panditrao MM, Rao S, Bajwa SJS, Sahay N, Tantry TP. Dissertation writing in post graduate medical education. Indian J Anaesth. 2022;66(1):34-46.
2. University of the People. (2024). Dissertation vs thesis: The differences that matter. [online] Available from https://www.uopeople.edu/blog/dissertation-vs-thesis/. [Last accessed July, 2025]
3. Fandino W. Formulating a good research question: Pearls and pitfalls. Indian J Anaesth. 2019;63:611-6.
4. Grewal A, Kataria H, Dhawan I. Literature search for research planning and identification of research problem. Indian J Anaesth. 2016;60(9):635-9.
5. Hall GM. Structure of a scientific paper. In: Hall MG (Ed). How to write a scientific paper, 3rd edition. Navarra: BMJ Publishing Group; 2003. pp. 6-15.
6. Harsoor SS. Art and science of authorship for biomedical research publication. Indian J Anaesth. 2016;60(9):679-83.

2

CHAPTER

Research Study Design

Laxmikant L

INTRODUCTION

Research study design is fundamental to scientific inquiry, providing a structured approach for investigating questions, testing hypotheses, and generating knowledge. The choice of study design affects the quality and reliability of the data influencing how findings are interpreted and applied. This chapter delves deeply into the definition of study design, variables, types of studies, and key considerations including observational and experimental designs as well as systematic reviews and meta-analyses and qualitative studies.[1,2]

DEFINITION

Study design refers to the systematic plan or methodology employed to conduct research, including how data is collected, analysed, and interpreted to answer a specific research question. The design dictates the structure of the study and the methods used, which in turn affect the validity, reliability, and generalisability of the results. A well-chosen study design ensures that the research question is addressed appropriately and that the conclusions drawn are based on robust evidence.[1,2]

Key aspects of study design include:

- *Purpose:* The overarching goal of the research, such as exploring a new phenomenon, testing a theory, or evaluating an intervention.
- *Methods:* The procedures used to gather and analyse data, including sampling techniques, data collection instruments, and statistical analyses.
- *Ethics:* Ensuring that the study is conducted with integrity and respect for participants, including obtaining informed consent and protecting confidentiality.

The choice of study design is critical because it impacts the ability to draw valid conclusions. A study design must be aligned with the research question, the type of data needed, and the resources available.

VARIABLES

Variables are measurable attributes that can vary among subjects or over time. Understanding variables is essential for designing a study and interpreting its results.

- *Variable:* Any characteristic or attribute that can be measured and can change or vary. Examples include age, sex, weight, health status, and test scores. Variables can be independent (exposures or interventions) or dependent (outcomes).
- *Exposure/intervention versus outcome:*
    - *Exposure/intervention:* Refers to the factor or condition being studied for its effects. In observational studies, exposures are naturally occurring, such as environmental or lifestyle factors (e.g., smoking and air pollution). In experimental studies, interventions are actively manipulated by the researcher (e.g., administering a new medication, changing a treatment protocol).

- *Outcome:* The result or effect that follows from the exposure or intervention. Outcomes can be health-related (e.g., disease incidence, mortality) or related to other aspects of interest (e.g., quality of life and behavioural changes).

Understanding these concepts is crucial for selecting appropriate measures and ensuring that the study design can accurately capture and analyse the relationships between variables.

TYPES OF STUDIES

Studies can be broadly categorised into observational and interventional/experimental designs, each serving different purposes and providing different types of evidence **(Table 1)**.[1-3]

Observational Studies

Observational studies involve monitoring and documenting naturally occurring relationships between exposures and outcomes without intervening. They are useful for exploring phenomena, generating hypotheses, and identifying patterns. However, they cannot establish causality due to the lack of control over variables.[4]

- *Descriptive studies:* These studies aim to summarise and describe data and characteristics of a population or phenomenon. They provide a factual account but do not infer causal relationships.
  - *Case reports:* Detailed descriptions of individual patients or small groups with specific conditions. They are useful for identifying new or rare conditions, unusual presentations, or potential adverse effects.
  - *Case series:* A collection of case reports involving patients with similar conditions, often drawn from one or more healthcare settings. Case series can highlight trends, common features, and potential areas for further research.
  - *Cross-sectional surveys:* Assess both exposure and outcome simultaneously in a population at a single point in time. They are useful for determining prevalence and understanding the current state of health or behaviour in a population. However, they cannot establish causality due to the simultaneous measurement of exposure and outcome.

TABLE 1: Types of studies and study designs.

Types	*Design*
Descriptive studies (observational): • Examine patterns of disease • Minimum ethical issues *Reach a hypothesis*	• Case reports • Case series • Cross-sectional study
Analytical studies (observational): • Studies of suspected causes of diseases • Comparison group, observation • Moderate ethical issue *Test hypothesis*	• Ecological study • Cross-sectional study • Case control • Cohort study • Nested case–control study • Case cohort
Experimental studies: • Compare treatment modalities • Comparison group, intervention • Serious ethical issues *Test hypothesis*	• Randomised control trials • Non-randomised control trials

Key questions:

1. Who has the disease?
2. What is the condition or disease being studied?
3. Why did the condition or disease arise?
4. Where does or does not the disease occur?

- *Analytical studies:* These studies test hypotheses and seek to determine causal relationships between variables. They are more complex than descriptive studies and include several key types.
    - *Case-control studies:* Compare individuals with a particular condition (cases) to those without the condition (controls) to identify potential risk factors or causes. This design is particularly useful for studying rare diseases or conditions. By comparing cases and controls, researchers can identify associations between exposures and outcomes.[5]
    - *Cohort studies:* Follow a group of individuals over time who are initially free of the outcome of interest. The cohort is divided based on exposure status, and the incidence of outcomes is observed. Cohort studies are valuable for assessing the temporal relationship between exposure and outcome and can provide information on incidence rates and risks.[6]
    - *Cross-sectional studies:* Measure both exposure and outcome at the same point in time, providing a snapshot of disease frequency and characteristics. They are useful for estimating prevalence and understanding associations but have limitations in establishing causality due to the simultaneous measurement of exposure and outcome.

Interventional (Experimental) Studies[1,2,7]

Interventional (experimental) studies involve the active manipulation of variables by the researcher to observe the effects of an intervention. These studies are designed to establish cause-and-effect relationships and are often considered the gold standard for evaluating interventions.

- *Randomised controlled trials (RCTs):* Participants are randomly assigned to either the intervention or control group. Randomisation helps to minimise biases and confounding variables, providing strong evidence for causality. RCTs are valuable for testing the effectiveness of new treatments, interventions, or therapies.
    - *Advantages:*
        - *Minimisation of bias:* Random allocation of participants helps to reduce selection bias and confounding factors.
        - *Blinding:* Participants and researchers can be blinded to the group assignments in order to minimise performance and detect biases.
        - *Strong evidence of causality:* The controlled environment and randomisation provide robust evidence of causal relationships.
    - *Disadvantages:*
        - *Cost and complexity:* RCTs can be expensive and logistically challenging to conduct.
        - *Ethical considerations:* Randomising participants to a control group may raise ethical issues, particularly if the intervention is believed to be beneficial.
- *Non-randomised controlled trials (Non-RCTs):*[8] A non-randomised experimental study, also referred to as a non-RCT or a non-experimental study, is one that does not utilise random assignment of participants to treatment groups. In these studies, participants may select the group they wish to join, or researchers may assign them to groups.

  Non-randomised studies are employed when random allocation is not feasible, such as in cases where RCTs present logistical or ethical challenges. However, these studies carry a higher risk of allocation bias compared to randomised studies because ensuring that treatment comparison groups are similar regarding prognostic variables can be challenging.

To address confounding in non-randomised studies, researchers may use methodological approaches such as:

- *Difference-in-differences:* This method compares changes in outcomes between locations that received the intervention and those that did not.

When conducting non-randomised studies, it is crucial to adhere to established data collection processes, including the use of a predefined data extraction template and dual extraction by two independent reviewers. Additionally, it is important to collect supplementary data to evaluate various types of biases.

Key considerations:

- *Observational studies:* Ideal for exploring phenomena and generating hypotheses. They are valuable for studying exposures and outcomes as they occur naturally but cannot confirm causation.
- *Interventional studies:* Provide strong evidence of causation through controlled experiments. They are useful for testing the effectiveness of interventions but can be complex and costly to conduct.

What is prospective and retrospective study design?[9]

Research designs are primarily categorised as prospective or retrospective. Prospective studies observe 'futuristic' outcomes of a population, while retrospective studies analyse outcomes which have already occurred, relying on past or historical data.

The term "prospective" reflects the future-oriented nature of these studies. Researchers select outcomes to measure in advance, then track these outcomes over time. This approach enhances the understanding of cause-and-effect relationships by linking outcomes to various study variables.

In contrast, "retrospective" studies determine the research question and methods beforehand but focus on analysing past data.

To clarify this further, consider a prospective study examining the link between smoking and lung cancer. Researchers would identify smokers and non-smokers, then follow them for several years to see if smokers develop lung cancer more frequently.

Retrospective studies, as their name suggests, look back in time, relying on existing data from past events. For example, a retrospective study might analyse historical records of lung cancer patients to determine the percentage of those who were smokers, thereby establishing a potential link.

One interesting type of prospective study is the combined retrospective and prospective study. This hybrid approach leverages data from past records while simultaneously collecting new forward-looking data. Such studies provide a richer dataset and a more comprehensive overview of a condition's incidence and progression.

For instance, a prospective observational study might involve researchers examining a diverse cross-section of the population over several years to assess how a specific lifestyle factor, such as diet or exercise, influences heart disease occurrence. This design allows researchers to draw meaningful conclusions about the relationship between lifestyle choices and heart disease within that population.

In summary, understanding these different research terminologies and concepts is crucial for conducting or interpreting studies. Whether a study is prospective, retrospective, cross-sectional, or longitudinal, each has unique strengths and limitations that need careful consideration.

Systematic Reviews and Meta-analyses[10,11]

The terms "systematic review" and "meta-analysis" are often used together, but they are distinct concepts and not interchangeable. While many systematic reviews incorporate meta-analyses, not all do.

Systematic Review

A systematic review is a thorough summary of all available evidence that meets predefined eligibility criteria to address a specific clinical question or set of questions. It follows a rigorous process that includes:

- Defining the research question, including study eligibility and methodology
- Systematically identifying studies that evaluate the specific research question(s)
- Critically appraising the studies
- Conducting meta-analyses (though this is not always performed)
- Presenting key findings, often in a summary of findings table
- Explicitly assessing the limitations of the evidence by rating the certainty (or quality) of the evidence base.

Systematic reviews differ from "narrative" reviews and textbook chapters, which typically do not conduct exhaustive literature reviews. Narrative reviews often lack transparency in evidence selection and interpretation, do not provide quantitative data synthesis, and may be biased if evidence is selectively chosen to support a predetermined conclusion instead of deriving conclusions from the entire body of evidence.

Meta-analysis

Meta-analysis, frequently included in systematic reviews, is a statistical method used to quantitatively combine or pool results from multiple studies. It provides overall pooled effect estimates. For example, if several placebo-controlled trials evaluate the same drug and report the same outcome, a meta-analysis can estimate a pooled relative risk for the drug's overall effect based on all trials. Meta-analysis can also aggregate other types of data, such as diagnostic accuracy studies (e.g., pooled estimates of sensitivity and specificity) and epidemiological studies (e.g., pooled incidence or prevalence rates and pooled odds ratios). Enhancements such as meta-regression and network meta-analysis build on traditional meta-analysis techniques.

Advantages of Systematic Review and Meta-analysis

Clinical decisions in medicine should ideally be guided by a comprehensive assessment of available knowledge. A single clinical trial, even if large, rarely provides a definitive answer to a clinical question. Indeed, analyses suggest that many research claims are later proven incorrect or inaccurate as more studies are conducted. Additionally, large RCTs do not always confirm the findings of previous meta-analyses. Understanding the "truth" requires a critical and objective examination of all data sources.

There are several potential benefits to conducting systematic analyses, including meta-analysis:

- Unique characteristics of a single randomised trial—such as the patient population, protocol, setting, or the expertise of the clinicians involved—may limit its generalisability to other contexts. Systematic reviews generally offer more generalisable conclusions than individual studies.
- Meta-analysis increases the sample size by combining studies, leading to more precise effect size estimates (with smaller confidence intervals) than those obtained from a single trial. It may also help explore reasons for variability

across studies, providing insights that go beyond what individual studies can reveal.

- Clinicians often lack the time or resources to critically evaluate all relevant evidence for a clinical question; systematic reviews facilitate this process.
- Unlike narrative reviews, which may selectively include studies chosen by the author, systematic reviews focus on narrowly defined questions and encompass all eligible studies. This comprehensive approach reduces bias, as conclusions are derived from the entire body of evidence.

Systematic reviews and meta-analyses synthesise available evidence using a transparent and explicit methodology that considers the strengths and weaknesses of individual studies, populations, interventions, and specific outcomes. Practitioners, policymakers, and guideline developers can rely on well-conducted systematic reviews to inform optimal patient management decisions. Organisations that create guidelines can utilise the findings from systematic reviews and meta-analyses to formulate evidence-based recommendations for care.

Qualitative Study Design

Qualitative study designs can be selected for various reasons, for instance, one might want to explore how nurses perceive or experience care in the intensive care unit, or one may seek to understand how individuals involved in heavy substance use feel about their interactions with a support agency. These designs are particularly useful for research questions aimed at gaining unique insights into specific contexts or social situations. However, they are less effective when the goal is to establish direct cause-and-effect relationships or to achieve statistically significant results.

Qualitative studies focus on understanding phenomena through in-depth exploration, Focused Group Discussion often using interviews, observations, and other non-numerical methods. They are valuable for discovering frameworks, generating theories, and gaining insights into complex issues.

Qualitative research focuses on gaining a deeper understanding of phenomena through interviews, observations and open-ended exploration, producing rich, descriptive, and subjective insights. It emphasises discovering new frameworks and generating theories. It prioritises the quality of participants over sample size. In contrast, quantitative research aims to measure, predict, and test theories using existing frameworks and numerical data collected through structured surveys or experiments. It values large, representative samples for reliability, seeks objectivity and generalisation, while relying more on statistical methods for analysis.[8]

CONCLUSION

Understanding research study designs is essential for conducting and interpreting scientific investigations effectively. The choice between observational, experimental, qualitative, or systematic review approaches depends on the research question, objectives, and available resources.. A well-selected and properly executed study design enhances the reliability, validity, and applicability of research findings.

REFERENCES

1. Ranganathan P, Aggarwal R. Study designs: Part 1–An overview and classification. Perspect Clin Res. 2018;9(4):184-6.
2. Grimes DA, Schulz KF. An overview of clinical research: The lay of the land. Lancet. 2002;359:57-61.
3. Grimes DA, Schulz KF. Descriptive studies: What they can and cannot do. Lancet. 2002;359:145-9.
4. Grimes DA, Schulz KF. Bias and causal associations in observational research. Lancet. 2002;359:248-52.

5. Schulz KF, Grimes DA. Case-control studies: Research in reverse. Lancet. 2002;359:431-4.
6. Grimes DA, Schulz KF. Cohort studies: Marching toward outcomes. Lancet. 2002;359:341-5.
7. Howick J. The philosophy of evidence-based medicine. Chichester, West Sussex, UK: Wiley-Blackwell, BMJ Books; 2011.
8. Jeremy H, Iain C, Paul G, Trish G, Carl H, Alessandro L et al. "The 2011 Oxford CEBM Evidence Levels of Evidence (Introductory Document)". Oxford Centre for Evidence-Based Medicine. Available from: https://www.cebm.ox.ac.uk/resources/levels-of-evidence/levels-of-evidence-introductory-document. [Last accessed July 2025]
9. Folia Health. Research Explainer Series: Prospective Outcomes Studies. [online] Available from https://www.foliahealth.com/study-designs. [Last accessed July, 2025]
10. Page MJ, McKenzie JE, Bossuyt PM, Boutron I, Hoffmann TC, Mulrow CD, et al. The PRISMA 2020 statement: an updated guideline for reporting systematic reviews. BMJ. 2021;372:n71.
11. Page MJ, Moher D, Bossuyt PM, Boutron I, Hoffmann TC, Mulrow CD, et al. PRISMA 2020 explanation and elaboration: updated guidance and exemplars for reporting systematic reviews. BMJ. 2021;372:n160.

CHAPTER 3

Preparing and Submitting a Synopsis

Maneesha Godbole

INTRODUCTION

Universities require students pursuing postgraduation, to undertake a research project. This is a requirement for obtaining the Masters/PhD degree. Preparing a synopsis of one's proposed research is the first step in this process.

WHAT IS A SYNOPSIS?

The word "Synopsis" has its origin in Greek—sun—together, opsis—seeing, meaning, a brief summary of something (Oxford English Dictionary).

Going through a synopsis, the reader should be able to get an overview of the research project.

It is a summary of the work one is going to undertake.

The purpose of writing a synopsis is:

- To register the project with the concerned university as requirement for obtaining one's degree.
- To obtain clearance from the ethical committee.
- To obtain approval from the institution to conduct the study.
- To obtain suggestions to help improve the research work, from the peer group or faculty.
- To obtain funding from different funding agencies.

Formats for a synopsis are provided by the university/institutions **(Annexure 6)**. In general, the structure of a synopsis should have the following parts:

- Title
- Introduction
- Statement of the problem, justification for undertaking the study and hypothesis
- Aims and objectives
- Review of literature
- Methodology—study design, sample size and selection of sample, data variables, data collection method, proposed analysis, and time frame
- References
- Official permission documents.

Title

This is like the main front cover of the entire work. Therefore, a lot of care should go into framing the title correctly—it should be brief but informative. Use of unnecessary adjectives should be avoided. It should neither be too short nor too long. Any name of the institution, the number of cases to be studied should not be included. The hypothesis to be studied can be included.

The title should be:

- Clear and concise
- Include keywords pertaining to the research topic
- Should convey the main objective, study design, population covered.
- Include the outcome being studied

"Exercise and heart health" is an example of a bad title. A better title would be:

"The impact of exercise on cardiovascular health in young adults—a longitudinal study".

Introduction

This should give a broad description of the subject of research, and its status in the world, country, and state. Statistical figures should be presented with due references. Introduction should be able to convey the importance of the topic that one is taking up for study.

Statement of the Problem or Hypothesis

The problem being studied should be mentioned in precise and clear terms. Understanding the problem aids the researcher in constructing the research proposal. It also allows the person to formulate the hypothesis. The problem under study should be relevant to the present time period. A brief account of its utility at the local or national level has to be discussed.

Hypothesis is mentioned as a tentative prediction or explanation of the relationship between two or more variables. Hypothesis should not be a haphazard guess but should be based on the existing knowledge and experience of the investigator. Hypothesis can be formulated by understanding the problem, reviewing the literature on it, and considering other factors. A researcher can state the problem and the hypothesis in about 200 words covering all the aspects described above. Usages of terms like "first study", "the only study", etc. should be avoided.

Aims and Objectives

All research projects should have objectives and aims and every effort should be made to achieve them. The objectives and aims should be only a few (2–3). They must pertain to the study problem.

Review of Literature

Review of literature is a very important part of a research project. It achieves the following:

- Familiarises the reader to the problem under study.
- It describes the work done by others either at local or international level on it or on a similar subject.
- It helps the researcher to understand the difficulties faced by others and the corrective steps taken or modifications made by them. The researcher can anticipate similar or additional problems during the study and review of literature helps him in anticipating them.
- Research methodology of the researcher can be structured and modified after reviewing the literature.
- The review assists in identifying various variables in the research project and conceptualises their relationship.
- Review of literature in a synopsis helps the reviewer in assessing the knowledge of the researcher. The reviewer can assess the work put in by the researcher and also assist in assessing the feasibility of the study.

The review of literature in a synopsis need not be exhaustive. The relevant information should be covered in about 300 words quoting 8–10 authentic, easily retrievable and recent references. Literature can be reviewed by using various scientific-information-gathering methods. These are journals, national, or international; bulletins of organisations such as World Health Organization (WHO), Centers for Disease Control and Prevention (CDC), and Indian Council of Medical Research (ICMR); books; computer-assisted searches such as Medline and Medlar; and personal communications with other researchers. Internet provides a vast avenue for information gathering. Care must be taken to retrieve only relevant information. In this era of information technology, review of literature is literally "just a click away".

Research Methodology

In a synopsis, the research methodology adopted should be mentioned in about 150–200 words. The research methodology forms the core of the research project. The methodology should cover the following aspects:

- Study design
- Study settings
- Sampling
- Variables
- Controls
- Study methods—examinations or investigations
- Data collection
- Data analysis
- Ethical clearance

Ethical Clearance

Wherever necessary, ethical committee clearance from the institute should be obtained, well in time for the last day of submission of the synopsis. The certificate must be attached. Ethical clearance is required in all human and animal studies.

Funding

There are some organisations or funding agencies that specifically provide funds for postgraduate research. Being prepared well in advance with the research question/topic will help one to tap into these opportunities. They will have their own requirement regarding the pattern of the proposal. So, in addition to the synopsis, one should be prepared with this.

References

All references quoted in review of literature and anywhere else in the synopsis should be listed. There are two styles for writing references, Vancouver style and Harvard style. Vancouver style is easy to follow as it depends on the numbers as quoted in text. However, the style as provided in the guidelines of the concerned University should be followed.

Official Requirements

A synopsis is incomplete if it does not contain the following information:

- Name of the researcher and designation
- Name and designation of the guide
- Name and designation of head of department/institution
- Name of the institution
- Signatures of all with official seal.

Synopsis writing is an important step in a research project. A good synopsis will give maximum information in minimum words. A well-conceived synopsis will go a long way in convincing the reviewer about the ability of the researcher to conduct the project. In cases of need for financial assistance, the request will be considered favourably. Thus, all research workers should make efforts to prepare a well-structured synopsis.

Acceptance/Rejection

After submitting the synopsis to the concerned authorities, it undergoes review by experts in the subject. In case of any lacunae, the synopsis is returned with comments to correct/modify certain points. After complying with the comments and necessary modifications, the synopsis has to be resubmitted. Once the acceptance is obtained, the process of data collection can be started. Submitting the proposal to various potential sources of funding can also be done once the synopsis is accepted.

Some Tips

One should always remember to have backup of the synopsis, at least in two places. This will save a lot of stress in case something goes wrong.

Falling into the trap of trying to gather a whole lot of data, just because one has a chance should be avoided. One should focus on the objectives and gather only relevant data.

Flowery language and adjectives should be avoided.

CONCLUSION

Preparing and submitting the synopsis is probably the most crucial step in postgraduate studies, that produces a lot of anxiety in the already stressed life of the student. Adequate knowledge about the steps involved in preparation of the synopsis, and good computer skills will make the process easier. A basic course in research methodology can be made mandatory, to make one eligible to join a postgraduate course. This would go a long way in improving the quality of postgraduate research work.

4

CHAPTER

Sample Size Estimation

Mahesh D Kurugodiyavar

INTRODUCTION

The quote *"In God we trust; all others must bring data"* by W Edwards Deming emphasises the importance of data in any field, especially research. It suggests that any statements or claims must be based on empirical evidence and researchers should base their decisions and conclusions on solid data rather than personal beliefs or assumptions. Without proper data-driven considerations, researchers risk drawing inaccurate conclusions or making faulty assumptions about the population being studied. When designing a research study, determining an appropriate sample size ensures that the results are reliable and meaningful. Understanding sampling and sample size is fundamental, and it is the bridge between the specific data we collect and the broader conclusions we aim to draw, impacting the validity and generalisability of our findings.

Sample size depends on the nature, scope, and type of the study which in turn are decided by the aim/objectives of the study. Hence only after the objectives have been clearly defined, a researcher can decide how large a sample to select from the population that is being studied.

BASIC STATISTICAL CONCEPTS[1,2]

The process of sample size estimation can be understood by first becoming familiar with basic statistical concepts.

Population versus Sample

The population refers to the entire group of individuals, items, or elements that share a common characteristic and are of interest to the researcher. It represents the larger group about which the researcher wants to make inferences or draw conclusions **(Fig. 1)**.

Suppose a researcher is interested in knowing duration of recovery from anaesthesia in a specific surgical procedure which can be summarised by various quantities, such as the mean (average duration), median (middle value for duration), mode (most common value for duration), and the variance (or standard deviation) which is a statistical measurement of the spread between various values for duration for this population. These quantities are called population parameters and are usually represented with *Greek letters*. It is not feasible or practical to study an entire population of patients undergoing this specific surgical procedure to know the true value of the population parameter, such as the mean duration due to limitations such as time, cost, and resources.

However, it is possible to estimate the true value with some degree of certainty (or uncertainty) from a random sample of patients undergoing this specific surgical procedure which is representative of the whole population and which reflects the true situation in the population. The estimates derived from this observed random

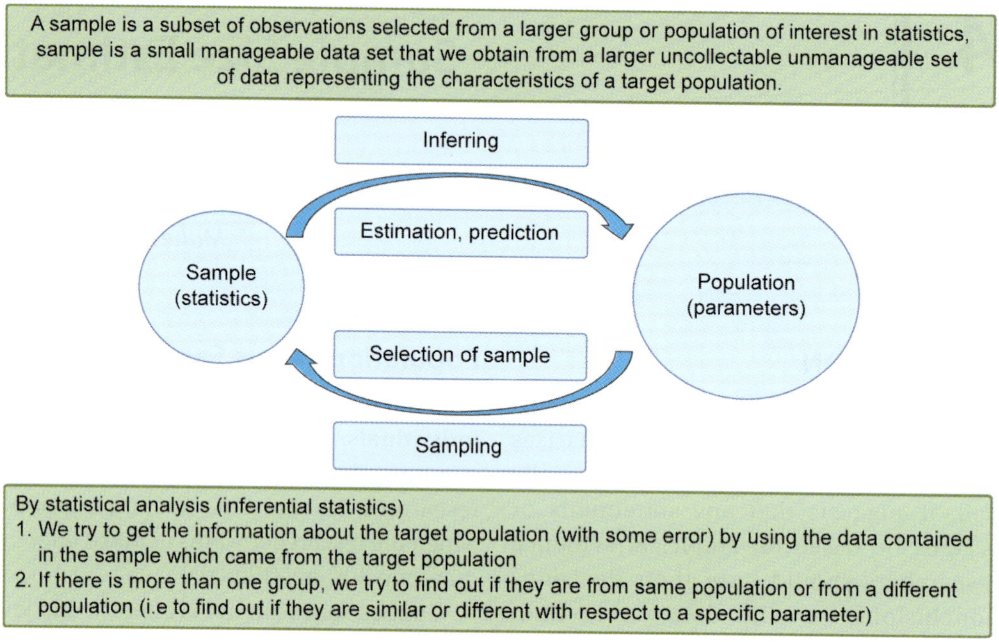

Fig. 1: Concept of sample and population.

TABLE 1: Notations used for population parameter and sample statistics.

Measure/observation	*Population parameter (Greek symbol)*	*Sample statistics (Roman/Latin letters)*
Number of cases	N	n
Mean	μ (Mu—population mean)	$\bar{x}$ (x bar)
Proportion	π (Pi—population proportion)	P (Sample proportion)
Standard deviation	σ (Sigma—population standard deviation)	s (Sample standard deviation)
Variance	σ^2 (Sigma square—population variance)	s^2 (Sample variance)
Correlation coefficient	ρ (Rho—population correlation coefficient)	r (Sample correlation coefficient)
Regression coefficient	β (Beta—population regression coefficient)	b (Sample regression coefficient)

sample are called sample statistics, and are denoted using *Roman/Latin letters* **(Table 1)**.

In some situations, the summary measure of interest may be a proportion (percent) rather than mean, for example, proportion of patients experiencing postoperative nausea and vomiting (PONV) after receiving a specific type of anaesthesia. This can be again estimated with some certainty (uncertainty) from a random sample of patients receiving a specific type of anaesthesia than the whole population.

Sampling Frame

Sampling frame is a source from which a sample will be selected. It is a list of all those within a population who can be sampled, and may include individuals, households, or institutions. For example, if we want to know the prevalence of anaemia among pregnant women, the population is the collection of all pregnant women. Sampling frame for a hospital-based study is all those pregnant women attending the antenatal clinic outpatient department of the hospital out of which the sample is selected. For a community-based study, the sampling frame is the list of all currently pregnant women residing in a defined geographical area **(Fig. 2)**.

Sampling Unit

It is the distinct and non-overlapping individual element (person, animal, or object) of a population which is considered for selection, that has the measurement (observation) taken in to the sample. In the above example, an individual pregnant woman is a sampling unit.

Alpha (α)

The significance level of a test: The probability of rejecting the null hypothesis when it is true (or the probability of making a Type I error).

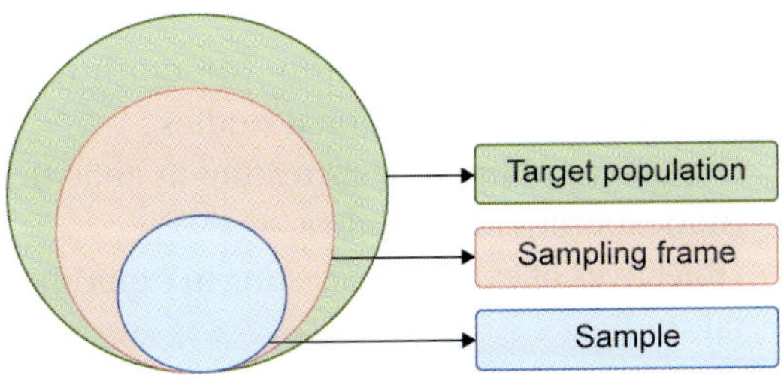

Fig. 2: Hierarchy of sampling.

Confidence Level

The probability that an estimate of a population parameter is within certain specified limits of the true value; commonly denoted by "1- α".

Beta (β)

The probability of failing to reject the null hypothesis when it is false (or the probability of making a Type II error).

Power

The probability of correctly rejecting the null hypothesis when it is false, denoted by "1–β".

Sampling Accuracy

It is a measure of the closeness of a sample-based parameter estimator to the true population value. When samples are representative (sample size is increased), sampling accuracy also increases. Rate of increase of sampling accuracy is very fast in the region of small samples and it slows beyond a certain sample size **(Fig. 3)**.

Sampling Precision or Margin of Error

This also is a measure of how close an estimate is to the true value of a population parameter, is related to the variability of the samples used, and determines the range of values that are expected to contain the true population values at a given probability. When the sample size

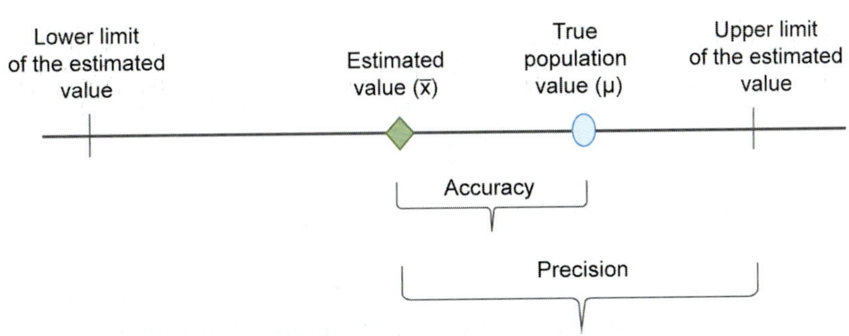

Fig. 3: Accuracy and precision.

increases, precision also increases as a result of decreasing variability. Margin of error is opposite of precision; lower the margin of error, higher will be the precision of the estimate.

Non-representativeness and small size of sample result in low accuracy and low precision.

Hence, if our results have to be accurate and highly precise:

- We should select a sample which is representative of the target population (using appropriate sampling techniques)
- We should have an adequate sample size

Determining the sample size is a very important issue because samples that are too large may waste resources without much gain in precision after a certain level, and may be unethical. Samples that are too small may lead to inaccurate and imprecise results.

Sample size determination may be done based on non-statistical considerations such as availability of resources, sampling frame, and sampling units without considering the expected level of precision or error in the final results and by statistical calculations based on prespecified level of precision and errors.

CALCULATION OF SAMPLE SIZE[3-6]

As mentioned before, sample size calculation can be done only after finalising the research objectives and hence one should be very clear about the objectives/research question. Sample size calculation in biomedical/health research requires some inputs based on what is being studied. It is better done taking the help of either a statistician with an ability to grasp the biomedical/clinical context of research, including familiarity with biomedical research designs and epidemiology or a biomedical researcher with good understanding of statistical theory and methods, including hypothesis testing.

Calculating Manually and by Using Software

Many computer software and mobile applications which are free (G-Power,[7] PS: Power and Sample Size Calculation[8]), open source (R software[9] with sample size packages), proprietary and commercial are available for sample size calculation. Some are online calculator tools. These applications and tools make the sample size calculation easy, especially when the calculations are complex and involve iterative process.

Sample size calculations can also be done using the standard recommended equations/formulas, the derivation of which is out of the scope of this book. Interested readers may refer to the standard books on sample size calculation.

Following are some very common broad categories of objectives of most of the biomedical/health research studies with examples and the equations used for manual calculation of sample size.

Objectives can be broadly classified in to the following:

- Objectives of estimation (of confidence intervals) in cross-sectional studies
- Objectives of hypothesis testing in analytical (nonexperimental) studies
- Objectives of hypothesis testing in experimental studies.

Objectives of Estimation (of Confidence Intervals)

Inputs required:

- Specification of a precision level
- Specification of level of confidence
- Specification of a population parameter based on:
    - Pilot studies
    - Results of previous studies/surveys
    - Own clinical experience and intelligent guess
    - Brainstorming with the peers/experts

Estimation of (Confidence Interval for) a Mean

Objective: To estimate the mean duration of postoperative pain relief provided by a specific analgesic medication.

$$n \geq \frac{(z_{1-\alpha/2})^2\sigma^2}{d^2}$$

For example, let us consider that it is known from previous studies that morphine provides postoperative analgesia for an average of 12–15 hours with a standard deviation of 3–4 hours.

Inputs required:

- d = 0.5 hours (precision level or margin of error)
- $z_{1-\alpha/2}$ = 1.96 (for 95% level of confidence)
- σ = 4 hours (population standard deviation for duration of analgesia of morphine from experience and previous studies)

$$n \geq \frac{(1.96)^2\, 4^2}{0.5^2} = 246$$

Considering population standard deviation for duration of analgesia of morphine as 4 hours, a minimum of 246 postoperative patients who received morphine are required to estimate the duration of postoperative analgesia with an error of ± 0.5 hours and with 95% confidence level.

Estimation of (Confidence Interval for) a Proportion

Objective: To estimate the proportion of patients experiencing intraoperative awareness under general anaesthesia (AAGA)

$$n \geq \frac{(z_{1-\alpha/2})^2\, P(1-P)}{d^2}$$

For example, let us consider that it is known from previous studies that cumulative incidence (incidence proportion) of AAGA is about 0.1–0.2%.

Inputs required:

- p = Proportion of patients experiencing AAGA = 0.002 (0.2%)

TABLE 2: Confidence level and the corresponding Z values.

Confidence level	$Z_{1-\alpha/2}$ *value*
0.999	3.29
0.998	3.09
0.995	2.81
0.99	2.57
0.98	2.33
0.95	1.96
0.90	1.64
0.80	1.28
0.50	0.67

- d = Precision level or margin of error = 0.0005 (0.05%)
- $z_{1-\alpha/2}$ = 1.96 (for 95% Level of confidence) **(Table 2)**

$$n \geq \frac{(1.96)^2\,(0.002)\,(0.998)}{0.0005^2} = 30671$$

Considering population proportion AAGA as 0.2%, a minimum of 30,671 subjects are required to estimate the cumulative incidence of AAGA with an error of ±0.05% and with 95% confidence level.

Note:

- *Observe that if the disease/condition or the outcome is rare, the sample size required would be large.*
- *p should always be in the form of proportion (not percent).*

Other Situations Where Objective is Estimation

- Difference between two independent means
- Difference between two paired means or proportions
- Area under the curve (AUC)
- Sensitivity and specificity
- Correlation coefficient

Objectives of Hypothesis Testing in Analytical (Non-experimental) Studies

Inputs required:

- Specification of alpha error
- Specification of beta error or power
- Specification of a population parameter

Hypothesis Testing for Two Independent Means (Cross-sectional Analysis within a Cohort Study)

Objective: To determine the association between smoking and mean blood pressure (BP)

Hypotheses:

- *Null hypothesis (H0):* There is no difference in mean blood pressure levels between smokers and non-smokers ($\mu_1 = \mu_2$).
- *Alternative hypothesis (H1):* There is a difference in mean BP levels between smokers and nonsmokers ($\mu_1 \neq \mu_2$).

$$n_1 = n_2 \geq \frac{(z_{1-\alpha/2} + z_{1-\beta})^2 \sigma^2}{(\mu_1 - \mu_2)^2}$$

n_1 = Sample size for smokers' group
n_2 = Sample size for non-smokers' group

Inputs required:
$Z_{1-\alpha/2}$ = Z table value for alpha error **(Table 3)**
$Z_{1-\beta}$ = Z table value for beta (power) **(Table 4)**
μ_1 = Mean BP in smokers
μ_2 = Mean BP in nonsmokers
σ = Pooled standard deviation

$$\sigma = \sqrt{\frac{\sigma_1^2 + \sigma_2^2}{2}}$$

σ_1 = Standard deviation for BP in smokers
σ_2 = Standard deviation for BP in non-smokers

Hypothesis Testing for Two Independent Proportions (Cohort or Prospective Studies)

Objective: To determine whether a demanding job is associated with an increased risk of developing cardiovascular disease.

TABLE 3: Alpha error and corresponding Z value.

Alpha error value	*$Z_{1-\alpha/2}$ value*
0.001	3.29
0.002	3.09
0.005	2.81
0.01	2.57
0.02	2.33
0.05	1.96
0.10	1.64
0.20	1.28
0.50	0.67

TABLE 4: Beta error and corresponding Z value.

Beta error value	*$Z_{1-\beta}$*
0.001	3.09
0.002	2.88
0.005	2.57
0.01	2.33
0.02	2.05
0.05	1.64
0.10	1.28
0.20	0.84
0.50	0.00

Hypotheses:

- *Null hypothesis (H0):* The proportion of individuals developing heart disease is the same for those with demanding jobs and those with less demanding jobs ($p_1 = p_2$).
- *Alternative hypothesis (H):* The proportion of individuals with heart disease is different between those with demanding jobs and those with less demanding jobs ($p_1 \neq p_2$).

$$n_1 = n_2 \geq \frac{2PQ(z_{1-\alpha/2} + z_{1-\beta})^2}{(P_1 - P_2)^2}$$

n_1 = Sample size for exposure group (demanding job)
n_2 = Sample size for non-exposure group (less demanding jobs)

Inputs required:

$Z_{1-\alpha/2}$ = Table values for alpha error

$Z_{1-\beta}$ = Table values for beta error (power)

P_1 = Proportion developing heart disease in demanding jobs

P_2 = Proportion developing heart disease in less demanding jobs

$$P = (\text{Pooled proportion}) = \frac{P_1 + P_2}{2}$$

$$Q = 1 - P$$

Hypothesis Testing for Two Independent Proportions (Case–Control Studies)

Objective: To determine whether a demanding job is associated with the development of cardiovascular disease.

Hypotheses:

- *Null hypothesis (H0):* The proportion of individuals in demanding jobs is same for those with heart disease (cases) and those without heart disease (controls) ($p_1 = p_2$).
- *Alternative hypothesis (H):* The proportion of individuals in demanding jobs is different between those with heart disease (cases) and without heart disease (controls) ($p_1 \neq p_2$).

$$n_1 = n_2 \geq \frac{2PQ(z_{1-\alpha/2} + z_{1-\beta})^2}{(P_1 - P_2)^2}$$

n_1 = Sample size for cases (heart disease)

n_2 = Sample size for controls (without heart disease)

Inputs required:

$Z_{1-\alpha/2}$ = Z score for alpha error

$Z_{1-\beta}$ = Z score for beta error (power)

P_1 = Proportion with demanding jobs among cases (with heart disease)

P_2 = Proportion with demanding jobs among controls (without heart disease)

$$P = (\text{Pooled proportion}) = \frac{P_1 + P_2}{2}$$

$$Q = 1 - P$$

Hypothesis Testing for Two Independent Correlation Coefficients (Analytical Cross-sectional Studies)

Objective: To compare correlation between body mass index (BMI) and BP among males and females.

Hypotheses:

- *Null hypothesis (H0):* The correlation between BMI and BP is same in males and females ($\rho_1 = \rho_2$).
- *Alternative hypothesis (H):* The correlation between BMI and BP is different in males and females ($\rho_1 \neq \rho_2$).

$$n_1 = n_2 \geq \frac{2(z_{1-\alpha/2} + z_{1-\beta})^2}{\left(0.5 \ln \frac{1+\rho_1}{1-\rho_1} - 0.5 \ln \frac{1+\rho_2}{1-\rho_2}\right)^2}$$

n_1 = Sample size for males

n_2 = Sample size for females

Inputs required:

$Z_{1-\alpha/2}$ = Z value for alpha error

$Z_{1-\beta}$ = Z table value for beta (power)

ln = Natural log

ρ_1 = Correlation coefficient in group 1 (males)

ρ_2 = Correlation coefficient in group 2 (females)

Other Situations where Objective is Hypothesis Testing

Table 5 highlights and summarises the commonly done study designs for which sample size calculations are done. Other studies where objective hypothesis testing are done include:

- Two paired means and proportions
- Two paired correlation coefficients
- More than two independent means
- More than two paired means (repeated measures)
- Two area under the curves (AUCs)

TABLE 5: Summary of sample size calculation situations.

Study design	*Objective*	*Examples*	*Required information from pilot/past studies*
• Case report • Case series • Pure descriptive	To explain a new condition	Clinical profile of a disease X	Sample size cannot be calculated (No generalisation)
Cross-sectional (survey)	Estimate (CI for) a proportion for one group	Proportion of patients having complications	Proportion (percentage) of variable which has to be estimated
	Estimate (CI for) a mean for one group	Average weight, blood glucose, Hb	SD for the variable for which mean has to be estimated
Analytical study: • Case control • Cohort • RCT	Comparison of proportion in more than one groups	Comparison of proportion of patients with complications between two surgeries	Proportion of variable in different groups
	Comparison of mean in more than one groups	Comparison of mean weight between males and females	Mean and SD of variable in different groups

(CI: confidence interval; Hb: haemoglobin; RCT: randomised controlled trial; SD: standard deviation)

Objectives of Hypothesis Testing in Experimental Studies: Outcome Variable is Continuous

Inputs required:

- Specification of alpha error
- Specification of beta error or power
- Specification of a population parameter:
    - Effect size
    - Clinical margins (superiority, noninferiority, equivalence)

Superiority Trial: To Demonstrate that a New Treatment is Better than an Existing Standard Treatment or Placebo

Objective: To determine whether a new drug (N) is superior to the standard drug (S) in improving cognitive function scores.

Hypotheses:

- *Null hypothesis (H0):* $\mu_N \leq \delta + \mu_S$ or $\mu_N - \mu_S \leq \delta$—

Drug N is not superior to drug S, i.e., mean increase in cognitive function score for drug N (μ_N) is lesser than or equal to mean increase in cognitive function scores for drug S (μ_S) by more than the superiority margin +δ.

- *Alternative hypothesis (H1):* $\mu_N > \mu_S + \delta$ or $\mu_N - \mu_S > \delta$—

Drug N is superior to drug S, i.e., mean increase in cognitive function score for drug N (μ_N) is greater than mean increase in cognitive function scores for drug S (μ_S) by more than the superiority margin +δ.

$$n_1 = n_2 \geq \frac{(z_{1-\alpha/2} + z_{1-\beta})^2 \sigma^2}{(\{\mu_N - \mu_S\} + \delta)^2}$$

Where,

$Z_{1-\alpha/2}$ = Z value for alpha error

$Z_{1-\beta}$ = Z table value for beta (power)

Superiority margin δ in superiority trial is generally taken as 0.

Noninferiority trial: To Demonstrate that a New Treatment is Not Worse than an Existing Treatment

Objective: To determine whether a new drug (N) is not worse than the standard drug (S) in improving cognitive function scores by more than a clinically acceptable margin (δ).

Hypotheses:

- *Null hypothesis (H0):* $\mu_N \leq \mu_S - \delta$ or $\mu_N - \mu_S \leq -\delta$

Drug N is *not noninferior* to standard drug S
[Mean cognitive function score for patients receiving the new drug N (μ_N) is less than or equal to the mean score for patients receiving the standard drug S (μ_S) by more than the noninferiority margin –δ].

- *Alternative hypothesis (H1):* $\mu_N > \mu_S - \delta$ or $\mu_N - \mu_S > -\delta$

Drug N is *noninferior* to drug S.
[Mean cognitive function score for patients receiving the new drug N (μ_N) is greater than the mean score for patients receiving the standard drug S (μ_S) by more than the noninferiority margin –δ].

The difference $\mu_N - \mu_S$ in noninferiority trial is generally taken as 0.

$$n_1 = n_2 \geq \frac{(z_{1-\alpha/2} + z_{1-\beta})^2\,\sigma^2}{(\{\mu_N - \mu_S\} + \delta)^2}$$

Equivalence Trial: To Demonstrate that a New Treatment is Therapeutically Similar to an Existing Treatment within a Prespecified Margin

Objective: To determine whether a new drug (N) is therapeutically equivalent to a standard drug (drug S) in terms of increasing cognitive function scores, within a specified equivalence margin (δ).

Hypotheses:

- *Null hypothesis (H0):* $|\mu_N - \mu_S| \geq \delta$ or ($\mu_N - \mu_S < -\delta$ or $\mu_N - \mu_S > +\delta$)—

Drug N is not equivalent to drug S, i.e., the absolute difference between the mean cognitive function scores for patients receiving the drug N (μ_N) and the branded drug S (μ_S) is greater than or equal to the equivalence margin δ.

- *Alternative hypothesis (H1):* $|\mu_N - \mu_S| < \delta$ or ($-\delta > \mu_N - \mu_S < +\delta$)—

Drug N is equivalent to drug S, i.e., the absolute difference between the mean cognitive function scores for patients receiving the drug N (μ_N) and the branded drug S (μ_S) is less than the equivalence margin δ.

$$n_1 = n_2 \geq \frac{(z_{1-\alpha/2} + z_{1-\beta})^2\,\sigma^2}{(\{\mu_N - \mu_S\} + |\delta|)^2}$$

These are the examples when the outcome variable is continuous and positive (higher the better). Similarly, when the outcome variable is continuous and negative (lower the better), these equations have to be appropriately modified.

Objectives of Hypothesis Testing in Experimental Studies: Outcome Variable is Proportion (Binary)

Inputs required:

- Specification of alpha error
- Specification of beta error or power
- Specification of a population parameter based on:
  - Effect size
  - Clinical margins (superiority, noninferiority, and equivalence)

Superiority Trial: To Demonstrate that a New Treatment is Better than an Existing Standard Treatment or Placebo

To test whether the proportion of patients cured (P_N) with new drug (drug N) is greater than the proportion of patients cured (P_S) with standard drug (drug S) or placebo by more than the superiority margin (δ).

$$n_1 = n_2 \geq \frac{(z_{1-\alpha/2} + z_{1-\beta})^2}{(\{P_N - P_S\} - \delta)^2}[P_N(1 - P_N) + P_S(1 - P_S)]$$

Noninferiority Trial: To Demonstrate that a New Treatment is not Worse than an Existing Treatment

To test whether the proportion of patients cured (P_N) with new drug (drug N) is greater than the proportion of patients cured (P_S) with standard drug (drug S) by more than the noninferiority margin (–δ).

$$n_1 = n_2 \geq \frac{(z_{1-\alpha/2} + z_{1-\beta})^2}{(\{P_N - P_S\} + \delta)^2}[P_N(1 - P_N) + P_S(1 - P_S)]$$

Equivalence Trial: To Demonstrate that a New Treatment is Therapeutically Similar to an Existing Treatment within a Prespecified Margin

To test whether the difference between proportion of patients cured with new drug and standard drug ($P_N - P_S$) is within the upper and lower equivalence margin (–δ to + δ).

Or

To test whether the absolute difference between proportion of patients cured with new drug and standard drug ($P_N - P_S$) is less the equivalence margin (δ).

$$n_1 = n_2 \geq \frac{(z_{1-\alpha/2} + z_{1-\beta})^2}{(\{P_N - P_S\} + |\delta|)^2}[P_N(1 - P_N) + P_S(1 - P_S)]$$

These are the examples when the outcome variable is binary (proportion) and positive (higher the better). Similarly, when the outcome variable is binary (proportion) and negative (lower the better), these equations have to be appropriately modified.

Sample Size Calculation or Power Analysis

Both, power calculation and sample size calculation are important concepts in research design.

Sample size calculation: Done to determine the number of participants (sample size) when one has a preliminary idea about the level of precision in the estimate that is needed to be achieved (or about the effect size and desired level of power that is needed to be achieved). This is done mainly for studies with objective of estimation of confidence interval.

Power calculation/analysis: Done to determine the power (probability of detecting a true statistically significant effect) once one has a better idea of the feasible sample size based on recruitment limitations. This is done while planning research studies with objective of testing the hypothesis.

Both power calculation and sample size calculation are crucial for designing a good research study; the most appropriate approach depends on the research question/research objective.

CONCLUSION

- Sample size calculation can be done manually or using computer applications.
- Sample size has to be calculated for the primary objective.
- If there are more than one primary objectives, sample size has to be determined for each objective and the higher sample size should be selected.

- Proper understanding of different types of biomedical data and basic statistical concepts is essential for determining sample size.
- Sample size calculation requires some inputs based on what is being studied.
- Final sample size should be more than the calculated to account for attrition, due to drop out, loss to follow up and for missing data.
- A clearly defined research problem/objective will help in proper planning of a research study including determination of appropriate sample size and gets the results with a minimum level of precision beyond which more precise results would not alter the intended action. On the other hand, the results of a research study with a poorly defined research problem/objective may be irrelevant even if the results are precise.

The renowned mathematician, John W Tukey has rightly said,

"An approximate answer to the right problem is worth a good deal more than an exact answer to an approximate problem".

REFERENCES

1. Daniel WW. Biostatistics: A Foundation for Analysis in the Health Sciences. United Kingdom: John Wiley & Sons (Asia) Pte, Limited. 2006.
2. Bellera CA, Foster BJ, Hanley JA. Calculating Sample Size in Anthropometry. In: Preedy, V. (ed) Handbook of Anthropometry. Springer, New York, NY. 2012:3-28.
3. Cohen J. Statistical power analysis for the behavioral sciences. 2nd ed. Hillsdale (NJ): Lawrence Erlbaum Associates; 1988.
4. Kishore K, Mahajan R. Understanding superiority, noninferiority, and equivalence for clinical trials. Indian Dermatol Online J. 2020;11(6):890-4.
5. Julious SA. Sample sizes for clinical trials. 2nd ed. Boca Raton (FL): Chapman & Hall/CRC Press; 2023.
6. Machin D, Campbell MJ, Tan SB, Tan SH. Sample sizes for clinical, laboratory and epidemiology studies. 4th ed. Hoboken (NJ): John Wiley & Sons; 2018.
7. Faul F, Erdfelder E, Lang AG, Buchner A. GPower [Computer program]. Version 3.1.9.7. Heinrich-Heine-Universität Düsseldorf; 2023. [Last accessed August, 2025]. Available from: http://www.gpower.hhu.de/.
8. Dupont WD, Plummer WD Jr. PS: Power and Sample Size Calculator [computer program]. Version 3.1.2. Nashville (TN): Vanderbilt University, Department of Biostatistics; 2014. Available from: https:// vbiostatps.app.vumc.org/ [Last accessed August, 2025].
9. R Core Team. R: A language and environment for statistical computing [computer program]. Version 4.4.1. Vienna (Austria): R Foundation for Statistical Computing; 2024. Available from: https://www.R-project.org/ [Last accessed August, 2025].

5

CHAPTER

Ethics in Research, Presentation before Ethics Committee, and Ethics Committee Approval

Ram S Kaulgud, Prithpal Singh Matreja, Harsha Hegde

INTRODUCTION

Research involving human participants must follow the four basic principles of autonomy (respect for persons), beneficence (do good), nonmaleficence (do no harm), and justice (equality).[1] All proposals submitted on social, biomedical, and behavioural science research for health which involves human participants, or their biological material or data, must be reviewed and approved by an appropriately constituted Ethics Committee.[1,2] The approval of the protocol of the proposed research study/clinical trial by the ethics committee is an important initial step of preparing the dissertation by a postgraduate student. The role of Ethics Committee is to safeguard the dignity, rights, safety, and well-being of all research participants at each step of the research. The Ethics Committee also ensures that the research methods should be scientifically sound and examines the ethical implications/aspects of the chosen research design or strategy.[1,3-8]

Each institution must have its own Ethics Committee that should be registered under Department of Health Research (DHR) for academic research and if the institution wants to conduct clinical trials, the ethics committee must be additionally registered with Central Drugs Standard Control Organization (CDSCO). If any institution does not have its own ethics committee, it can utilise the services of the ethics committee of another institution or Institutional Review Board (IRB) provided the said committee/board is within the radius of 50 km from the host institution.[5,9]

SIGNIFICANCE OF ETHICAL COMMITTEE APPROVAL IN RESEARCH STUDIES

Halse, in 2011, defined Ethics Committee as a regime of power designed to control researchers by compelling them to conduct their research according to the norms, practices, and protocols or principles approved by institutional, state, and/or national guidelines. He also stated that the purpose of ethics review as a disciplinary system is to impose specific performative demands that discipline researchers and correct deviant behaviour so that the researchers conduct themselves according to sanctioned standards.[9,10]

NECESSITY OF ETHICS COMMITTEE APPROVAL[1,2,5,9]

- An interventional clinical trial cannot be initiated without prior approval of Institutional Ethics Committee (IEC).
- All the clinical trials are continuously monitored by the IECs, with regard to consent, protection of patient rights, conduct of study procedures, occurrence of serious adverse events (SAEs), and to make sure patients are adequately compensated if SAEs occur.

- IECs monitor conformation of researchers to good clinical practices (GCPs).
- It is now mandatory for any researcher to have approval of the IEC for applying for grants to any funding agency in India.
- IECs also make sure that academic integrity is maintained in research conducted within and also between different institutions.
- Obtaining IEC approval indicates that the researcher has accepted to adhere to the standards of genuine research.
- Participants have the right to know who has access to their data and what is being done with it.

COMPOSITION OF ETHICS COMMITTEE (FIG. 1)

The Ethics Committee is constituted by the Head of the Institution who will not be a part of the Ethics Committee, although the Head of the Institution can be an appellant. The committee will include members from multiple disciplines and multiple sectors with adequate representation of age and gender. At least half of the members in the ethics committee will be nonaffiliated to the institution.

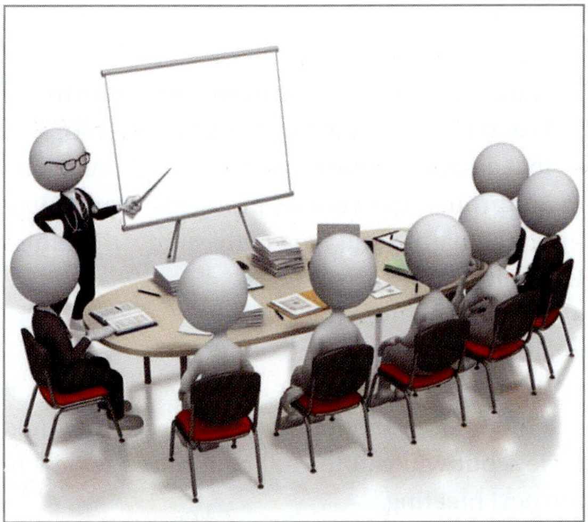

Fig. 1: Presentation before the Ethics Committee.

The number of members can vary from seven to fifteen and there will be a balance between medical and non-medical members—Chairperson/ Vice Chairperson, Member Secretary, Basic Medical Scientist, Clinician, Legal Experts, Social Scientist/Philosopher/Ethicist, Layperson. The Chairperson of the ethics committee will not be affiliated to the institution and the member secretary will be a person who will be able to devote time for the Ethics Committee.[1,2,3,9]

All the members of the Ethics Committee undergo certificate training on human research protection and guidelines on GCP with certificate, the same has to be submitted within 6 months of appointment. They further undergo training or update their skills and are aware of the relevant guidelines and regulations pertaining to the region in which the Ethics Committee is located. All members will be committed and willing to place their affiliation and sign an agreement on confidentiality and conflict of interest. The Ethics Committee members are well versed with the functions of the committee and standard operating procedures (SOPs) and are aware of the local, social, and cultural norms and emerging ethical issues.[4,9,11]

ROLES AND RESPONSIBILITIES OF ETHICS COMMITTEE

The Ethics Committee ensures that the rights, safety, dignity, and well-being of the research participants are protected and the research is conducted ethically. There are instances when a member of the Ethics Committee may also be a researcher for the study; in this scenario, the conflict of interest should be declared to the chairperson and the said member should abstain from the final decision process of the research protocol. The function of the Ethics Committee does not end with the grant of initial approval of the research proposal; the Ethics Committee continues the review of all ethical, medical, social, and scientific aspect of the proposal at appropriate intervals of time as mentioned in the SOP. The Ethics Committee ensures that universal ethical values and international scientific standards are followed throughout the research. The Ethics Committee also assists in development and education of research in the community and ensures the maintenance of privacy of the individual and confidentiality of data. The Ethics Committee carries out monitoring visits at the site and also reviews the progress report and final report of the proposal, any SAEs reported and provides needful suggestions. The committee recommends appropriate compensation for any injury related to research and discourages replicative research.[1,3,6,9]

The synopsis/protocol of the planned research study is submitted to the Ethics Committee in advance. This is followed by a formal meeting of the Ethics Committee members where the researcher/student orally presents the protocol with the help of PowerPoint **(Fig. 1)**. The protocol must have the following components:[6,8,9]

- The face page carrying the title of the proposal with signatures of the investigators
- Brief summary/lay summary
- Background with rationale of why a human study is needed to answer the research question
- Details of regulatory approval obtained in case of clinical trials
- Justification of inclusion/exclusion of vulnerable populations
- Clear research objectives and end points (if applicable)
- Eligibility criteria and participant recruitment procedures
- Detailed description of the methodology of the proposed research, including sample size (with justification), type of study design (observational, experimental, pilot, randomised, blinded, etc.), types of data collection, intended intervention, dosages of drugs, route of administration, duration of treatment, and details of invasive procedures, if any
- Duration of the study
- Justification for placebo, benefit–risk assessment, plans to withdraw. If standard therapies are to be withheld, justification for the same
- Procedure for seeking informed consent forms in English and local languages. Audiovisual recording if applicable; informed consent for stored samples
- Plan for statistical analysis of the study
- Plan to maintain the privacy and confidentiality of the study participants
- For research involving more than minimal risk, an account of management of risk or injury
- Proposed compensation, including details of the clinical trial insurance, reimbursement of incidental expenses and management of research-related injury/illness during and after the research period
- Provision of ancillary care for unrelated illness during the duration of research
- An account of storage and maintenance of all data collected during the trial
- Ethical considerations and safeguards for protection of participants.

The documents should be submitted sufficiently in advance to the Ethics Committee so that adequate time is available for all members to go through the various protocols. Depending upon the nature and type of the study, the Ethics Committee can go for:

- Exemption from review
- Expedited review
- Full committee review

The Ethics Committee may give an expedited review but will call for full committee review in the next meeting.[1]

Institutional Ethics Committee Format for Approval of Clinical Trial[2,6,9]

To,

(Name of Principal Investigator)

Subject: ______Ethics Committee approval of Clinical trial

Study Code:________

Study Title:________

Dear Dr.
We have received from you the copies of the following documents with reference to the letter

Dated ________ for conducting the clinical trials

IEC submission dossier contains following documents:

Sl. No. Study Documents

1. Curriculum Vitae (CV) of Principal Investigator (PI), Medical Registration Certificate of PI, Good Clinical Practice (GCP) Training Certificate of PI
2. Investigator's Undertaking (IU)
3. Protocol Signature Page (PSP)
4. Protocol Version
5. Investigator's Brochure
6. Master Informed Consent Form (ICF) Version No.
7. Drugs Controller General of India (DCGI) Approval letter ___ Version
8. Insurance (Period of Insurance)
9. Draft of Clinical Trial Agreement
10. Electronic Case Report Form (eCRF)___ Version (If Applicable)

At the Institutional Ethics Committee meeting held on __________ at ______ in ________ (Institute name), the above-mentioned documents were examined, reviewed, and discussed. The details of members who attended the meeting are as follows:

Sl. No.	*Name and qualification*	*Affiliation to the institute*	*Title*	*Present/absent*

We approve the protocol, investigator brochure, and other study-related documents submitted in its presented form.

We hereby confirm that neither you nor any of your study team members have participated in the voting/decision making procedure of the committee. The members of the committee who have participated in the voting/decision-making procedure of the committee do not have any conflict of interest in the referenced study.

The Institutional Ethics Committee, ________ expects to be informed about:

1. The progress of the study annually
2. Any serious adverse event (SAE) occurring in the course of the study
3. Any changes in the protocol and patient information/informed consent

Also, you are requested to provide a copy of the final report.

The Ethics Committee is organised and operates according to Good Clinical Practice, ICMR, and all other applicable requirements in accordance with The New Drugs and Clinical Trials Rules, 2019.

The Ethics Committee is registered with the DCGI with the registration number __________

Yours sincerely,
Chairperson/Member secretary,___________Ethics committee

WHAT IS GOOD CLINICAL PRACTICE?[4,6]

It is an international ethical and scientific quality standard for designing, conducting, performing, monitoring, recording, analysing, and reporting of clinical trials that involve the participation of human subjects. It provides assurance that the data and reported results are credible and accurate and that the rights, integrity, and confidentiality of the trial subjects are protected. Some of the principles include the following:

- Clinical trials should be conducted in accordance with the ethical principles that have their origin in the Declaration of Helsinki.
- A trial should be initiated and continued only if the anticipated benefits justify the risks.
- The rights, safety, and well-being of the trial subjects are the most important considerations.
- The available clinical and nonclinical information on an investigational product should be adequate to support the clinical trial.
- A trial should be conducted in compliance with the protocol that has received institutional review board/institutional ethics committee approval.
- The medical care given to, and medical decisions made on behalf of subjects should always be the responsibility of a qualified physician.
- Each individual involved in conducting a trial should be qualified by education, training, and experience.
- Freely given informed consent should be obtained from every subject before participation in the clinical trial.
- All clinical trial information should be recorded, handled, and stored in a way that allows its accurate reporting, interpretation, and verification.
- The confidentiality of patient records and the privacy of patients should be protected.
- Investigational products should be manufactured, handled, and stored in accordance with applicable good manufacturing practice.

ETHICAL ISSUES RELATED TO REVIEWING OF PROTOCOL[1,3,5,11]

- Social values
- Scientific design and conduct of the study
- Benefit–risk assessment
- Selection of the study population and recruitment of research participants
- Payment for participation
- Protection of research participants' privacy and confidentiality
- Community considerations
- Qualifications of researchers and adequacy assessment of study sites
- Disclosure or declaration of potential conflict of interest
- Plans for medical management and compensation for study related injury
- Review of the informed consent process

TYPES OF DECISIONS OF THE ETHICS COMMITTEE[1,5]

- Approved/favourable opinion
- Revision with minor modifications/amendments
- Revision with major modifications for resubmission
- Not approved/negative opinion
- Termination/suspension of any prior approval/favourable opinion

REASONS FOR REJECTION OF SYNOPSIS BY ETHICS COMMITTEE[6,11]

The IEC may reject a synopsis submitted by a postgraduate student. This may be due to several reasons.

- *Novelty:* The study is a replication of recent research conducted by another researcher from the same university.

- *Vulnerable population:* Any intervention study involving the vulnerable population groups such as pregnant women, infants, and mentally challenged subjects carries high chances of rejection by the IEC. Exceptions are studies aiming to improve quality of life or outcomes and carrying minimum risks.
- *Novel therapy:* Studies which involve therapies for diseases which have not been accepted as standard of care are rejected. Examples include using drugs for indications other than they have been approved, study of drugs which are still not in market, and using drugs whose benefit is questionable from the presently available literature.
- *Study design:* The study design should conform to the standards of research. Gross deviations will lead to rejection of study.
- *Procedural risks:* Studies carrying significant procedural risks are likely to be rejected. Examples include carrying out lumbar puncture or bone marrow biopsy for study purpose only, though they are not strictly indicated as per existing standards of practice.
- *Care facilities:* If in a study, there is a possibility of a medical emergency developing and the hospital does not have the emergency care facilities, the study will be rejected.

REAPPLICATION TO ETHICS COMMITTEE[11]

- The reason for initial rejection is the primary factor that decides when to reapply to the Ethics Committee.
- If the concept of the study was rejected, then modification is needed before applying again for approval. The student can reapply with modifications.
- If defective objectives are the reason for rejection, correction is essential before reapplying.
- If there is potential risk to the participants, the student will have to make essential changes in the study so that the concerns of the Ethics Committee are addressed.
- If the study design is not correct, one can reapply for approval after making necessary changes.
- The studies requiring regulatory approval are not accepted as a part of postgraduate dissertation.
- If the study is rejected for lack of novelty, changes in the title and design of the study are necessary before applying again.
- If the study is rejected because of lack of care facilities, it cannot be conducted till such facilities are developed within the institute.

MONITORING OF RESEARCH BY ETHICS COMMITTEE[4,6,9]

The Ethics Committee monitors and supervises the progress of research proposal and any deviation/change in protocol must be reported to the committee and fresh approval should be sort for all amendments done. The ethics committee might give a call of *"for cause" monitoring* in certain situations:

- High number of protocol violations/deviations
- Large number of proposals carried out at the study site or by the same researcher
- Large number of SAE reports
- High recruitment rate
- Complaints received from participants
- Any adverse media report
- Adverse information received from any other source
- Non-compliance with Ethics Committee directions
- Misconduct by the researcher
- Any other cause as decided by the Ethics Committee.

CONCLUSION

All research proposals on biomedical, social and behavioural science involving human participants, their biological material and data need to be reviewed and approved by an appropriately constituted IEC. The approval by the committee is essential for initiating studies and securing research grants. The committee confirms whether the adopted research methods in the study are scientifically sound, and examines the ethical implications of the chosen research design or strategy. Rejections may occur due to risks, design flaws, or lack of novelty, but researchers can reapply with modifications. The main role of the Ethics Committee is to safeguard the dignity, rights, safety and well-being of all the research participants and foster responsible and credible research.

REFERENCES

1. Indian Council of Medical Research. (2017). National ethical guidelines for biomedical research involving human participants. [online] Available from https://ethics.ncdirindia.org/asset/pdf/ICMR_National_Ethical_Guidelines.pdf. [Last accessed July, 2025]
2. International Council for Harmonisation of Technical Requirements for Pharmaceuticals for Human Use (ICH). (2016). ICH Harmonised Guideline - Integrated Addendum to ICH E6(R1): Guideline For Good Clinical Practice - E6(R2). [online] Available from https://database.ich.org/sites/default/files/E6_R2_Addendum.pdf. [Last accessed July, 2025]
3. Indian Council of Medical Research. (2006). Ethical Guidelines for Biomedical Research on Human Participants. [online] Available from https://ethics.ncdirindia.org/asset/pdf/ICMR_National_Ethical_Guidelines.pdf. [Last accessed July, 2025]
4. Clinical Net. 13 Principles of Good Clinical Practice. [online] Available from https://www.clinicalnet.com/13-principles-of-good-clinical-practice/. [Last accessed July, 2025]
5. Indian Council of Medical Research. (2018). Handbook on National Ethical Guidelines For Biomedical Research Involving Human Participants by ICMR. [online] Available from https://naitik.gov.in/DHR/resources/app_srv/DHR/global/pdf/downloads/Handbook_on_ICMR_Ethical_Guidelines.pdf. [Last accessed July, 2025]
6. International Council For Harmonisation of Technical Requirements for Pharmaceuticals For Human Use. (2023). ICH Harmonised Guideline - Good Clinical Practice (GCP) - E6(R3). [online] Available from https://database.ich.org/sites/default/files/ICH_E6%28R3%29_DraftGuideline_2023_0519.pdf. [Last accessed July, 2025].
7. U.S. Department of Health And Human Services, Food And Drug Administration. (2023) Informed Consent - Guidance for IRBS, Clinical Investigators, And Sponsors. [online] Available from https://www.fda.gov/regulatory-information/search-fda-guidance-documents/informed-consent?utm_medium=email&utm_source=govdelivery. [Last accessed July, 2025].
8. Indian Council of Medical Research. (2017). National Ethical Guidelines For Biomedical Research Involving Children. [online] Available from https://www.researchgate.net/publication/380636964_National_Ethical_Guidelines_for_Biomedical_Research_Involving_Children?channel=doi&linkId=6646d95e0b0d2845743b8312&showFull. [Last accessed July, 2025].
9. Ministry of Health and Family Welfare, Government of India. (2019). New Drugs And Clinical Trials Rules, 2019. [online] Available from https://cdsco.gov.in/opencms/export/sites/CDSCO_WEB/Pdf-documents/NewDrugs_CTRules_2019.pdf. [Last accessed July, 2025].
10. Behera SK, Das S, Xavier AS, Selvarajan S, Anandabaskar N. Indian council of medical research's national ethical guidelines for biomedical and health research involving human participants: The way forward from 2006 To 2017. Perspect Clin Res. 2019;10:108-14.
11. National Institute Of Epidemiology Chennai. (2021). Institutional Human Ethics Committee - Standard Operating Procedures - Version 03.0 (1st October 2021). [online] Available from https://nie.gov.in/images/pdf/SOP_030_version_01102021.pdf. [Last accessed July, 2025].

6

CHAPTER

Clinical Trials Registry of India Registration

Milon V Mitragotri, Manoj Kumar

INTRODUCTION

Clinical Trials Registry-India (CTRI) is a nonprofit voluntary organisation set up by the Indian Council of Medical Research (ICMR) and National Institute of Medical Statistics (NIMS) launched in 2007 **(Flowchart 1)**. It was initiated as a part of a global endeavour to bring transparency, accountability, and accessibility of clinical trials wherein many registries have been established. Some common queries of students and researchers regarding study registration are addressed in this chapter.

Q1. Why do I need to register my trial in CTRI?

Ans:

- To make the general public aware of your study and to provide an opportunity to voluntarily be part of your study population. For example, during the coronavirus disease (COVID)-19 pandemic, many studies were registered, and the same information was available to the public.[1]
- To inform the medical fraternity as well as the public of the ongoing study and uprise them of the developments with regards to the study.
- Mandatory step as per Drugs Controller General of India (DCGI).
- Editors of major journals in India and abroad compulsorily seek CTRI registry number prior to publication.

Flowchart 1: Different trial registries of the world.

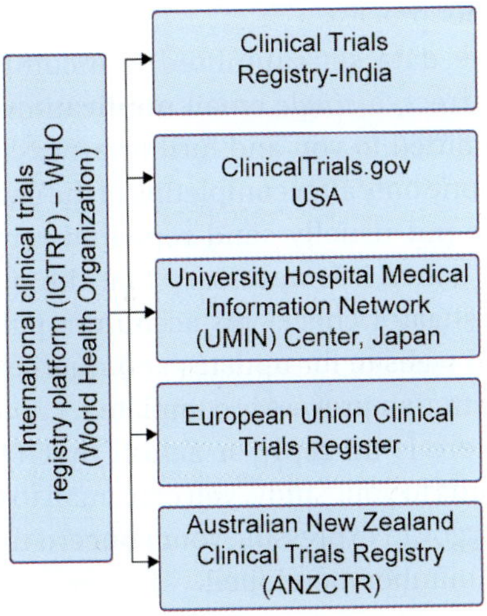

(USA: United States of America)

Q2. Do you need to register a postgraduate (PG) thesis?

Ans: Yes. It is necessary to register PG thesis for further publication and as per norms.

Q3. How do I register my trial?

Ans: CTRI registration is an online, hassle-free process done on the website www.ctri.nic.in and does not incur any cost. Creating an account in the name of the principal investigator on the website is the first step followed by registering of the trial.[2]

Q4. What are the essential details that I should know prior to registering my study?

Ans:

- All types of studies including observational, interventional, and analytic studies are accepted. However, it is necessary that the trial *is registered prior to recruiting your first patient.* Even retrospective studies are accepted for registration but the data collection should be started after trial registration.

- Trials should be submitted 15-20 days before the date of first enrolment to CTRI to allow time for review, trial modification, and receipt of email confirmation from trial contact persons.
- Prior to registration, make sure you have a pdf copy of the Ethics Committee approval letter for the said study in the prescribed standard format.
- It is not necessary to register the trials in multiple registers, e.g., ClinicalTrials.gov but if the trial is a part of a multicentric trial and India is one of the places of the study, it should be registered in CTRI adding the secondary identity document (ID) of ClinicalTrials.gov.
- The following data are asked during the registration process and should be known before proceeding for registration:
  - Public title of study
  - Scientific title of study
  - Secondary IDs—if also registered elsewhere
  - Principal investigator's (the PG student) name and address
  - Contact person for queries (Public query: PG student; Scientific query: PG guide)
  - Sources of monetary or material support
  - Primary sponsor (usually the college and hospital)
  - Secondary sponsor (usually nil in a PG thesis)
  - Countries of recruitment
  - Site/s of study
  - Name of ethics committee and approval status
  - Regulatory clearance obtained from DCGI (needed if using a new drug or using an old drug for new purpose)
  - Health condition/problem studied
  - Intervention and comparator agent
  - Key inclusion/exclusion criteria
  - Method of generating randomisation sequence
  - Method of allocation concealment
  - Blinding and masking
  - Primary outcome/s
  - Secondary outcome/s
  - Status of trial
  - Phase of trial
  - Study type
  - Date of first enrolment
  - Estimated duration of trial
  - Target sample size
  - Brief summary

Q5. How long does it take to complete the registration process?

Ans: The usual process of registration takes 7-10 days unless the details submitted are incomplete or incorrect. An email is sent to the principal investigator regarding the completion of registration process with registered number. For example, CTRI/2018/01/011621.

- Kindly note that getting a reference number such as REF/2017/01/013201 does not indicate completion of registration process. It is only an acknowledgement number for the further process.
- If the data set submitted is incomplete or incorrect, a *single* email notification will be submitted to you and further processing will be done only after completing of the data. CTRI does not usually send repeated reminders and hence it is necessary that the principal investigator checks his account regularly on CTRI website for updates and queries till the registration process is completed.
- If there is no reply or action by CTRI with regards to your study, you can email to CTRI at ctri@gov.in expressing your concern using the REF number mentioned.

Q6. What are the common causes of delay in the registration process?

Ans:

- Trial data uploaded but not yet submitted—if there is no issue of REF number, your article has not yet been submitted. Ensure you receive a REF number.
- Ethics/DCGI approval letter not uploaded.
- Non-receipt of verification email.
- Trial modifications needed.

Q7. I have registered my trial and want to modify the study design. Is it possible in the later part of the trial?

Ans: Yes. This can happen in case mistakes are found in the methodology during synopsis review and modifications are suggested by the synopsis reviewer. Some of the details of the trial are modifiable after following standard operating procedure (SOP) as prescribed by CTRI. Most of the details of the study design are locked and are not modifiable.

Q8. I have received my CTRI registration number. What to do next?

Ans:

- Start recruiting the cases for your study. Quote the CTRI registration number and Ethics Committee registration number in the material and methods section during the publication process. Few journals have separate buttons on their website to mention CTRI registration number.
- After the completion and publication of the study, make sure you update the CTRI website regarding the same. Even if the study is terminated or suspended, the same should be updated on the website. As per the Joint Statement of the World Health Organization (WHO) released in 2017 and endorsed by ICMR, all interventional trials would have to declare summary results within 1 year of trial completion. As per the Joint Statement of the WHO released in 2017 and endorsed by ICMR, all interventional trials would have to declare summary results within 1 year of trial completion.

Q9. What is prospective and retrospective registration of a study? Should registration always be prospective? Can it be retrospective?

Ans: The study is said to be prospectively registered if the enrolment of the first participant begins after the registration number is received. The study is retrospectively registered if the study is registered after the enrolment of one or more study participants. Prospective registration is ideal and mandatory for most studies published in medical journals because it provides transparency, protects study participants and prevents publication bias by providing a public record of the study.

CONCLUSION

The CTRI plays a paramount role in ensuring transparency, accountability and accessibility of clinical research in the country. Mandatory registration of all clinical trials, including PG theses, ensures this purpose. CTRI registration is a smooth sailing process when the principal investigator makes a well-prepared submission, complete with ethical approvals and accurate trial details.

REFERENCES

1. Rao MVV, Juneja A, Maulik M, Adhikari T, Sharma S, Gupta J, et al. Emerging trends from COVID-19 research registered in the Clinical Trials Registry - India. Indian J Med Res. 2021;153(1 & 2):26-63.
2. ctri.nic.in. New Delhi: Clinical Trials Registry-India. [Online] Available from http://www.ctri.nic.in/ (Last accessed July, 2025).

7 CHAPTER

Dissertation Writing – Title, Introduction, Aims and Objectives, Review of Literature, Abstract, References and Citation Management

Madhuri S Kurdi, Prashant Joshi

INTRODUCTION

The dissertation has to be written in a well-structured manner with some specific headings. The initial headings include title, abstract, introduction, aims and objectives, and review of literature. The title, aims and objectives are clearly written in the synopsis that is presented before the start of the research project of the dissertation. These will remain the same in the dissertation. The review of literature will be written in brief in the synopsis, whereas it will be written in detail in the dissertation.

This chapter touches upon the intricacies and finer aspects of framing the title, aims and objectives, writing sections of the dissertation such as the abstract, introduction, review of literature, references and also on how to do citation management.

THE TITLE

The title for the thesis is what an opening batsman is for a cricket match. It is the signpost of the study. The title should have the following characteristics:

- Should neither be too short and cryptic, nor should it be too long.
- Should be clear and brief.
- Should grab the readers' attention.
- Should be accurate with no spelling mistakes.
- Should be concise, descriptive, and informative.
- Should convey important content of the study.
- Should be specific and mention the type of study.
- Should not be misleading.
- Should not contain nonstandard abbreviations.
- Should reflect the purpose of the study.
- Should be scientific and not appear poetic.
- Should not be put in inverted commas.

Examples of well-framed titles of a research study are:

- *Comparison of ease of intubation with Airtraq®, Miller, Macintosh laryngoscope blades in children: A prospective randomised trial*
- *A randomised controlled trial comparing video laryngoscopy versus conventional blind technique for transoesophageal echocardiography probe insertion in paediatric patients undergoing cardiac surgery: A pilot study*

Examples of badly framed titles of a research study are:

- *To compare the efficacy of three techniques in reducing etomidate-induced myoclonus: A randomised controlled trial*
- *Transnasal humidified rapid insufflation ventilatory exchange (THRIVE): A game changer in apnoeic anaesthesia for shared airway procedures: A retrospective study*
- *Comparison of i-gel®, Ambu® AuraGain™, Baska Mask, LMA® Protector™ for airway management of obese surgical patients: A randomised comparative study.*

THE ABSTRACT SECTION

It is a summary of the study. It is like the icing on the cake. It is the first heading to be encountered by the reader and just like any "first look", it gives a general idea to the examiner regarding the study. It contains only important information related to the study. It is structured and written using subheadings such as Background, Objectives, Materials and Methods, Results and Conclusion. It will not contain discussion and references. Only important observations will be clearly indicated in it. *p* values and confidence intervals should be mentioned in the results. The present tense is used only for facts already established, especially in the background part. The past tense is used for parts already established or for findings of the study that the dissertation is based on. An abstract cannot be too long. The number of words is usually restricted to around 250–300.

THE INTRODUCTION SECTION

This is the first heading of the thesis that appears immediately after the table of contents. It should include the topics of the research/thesis, the focus and scope of the topic, and the aims of the research. The researcher makes the first connection with the reader through the introduction and hence it should be written in a manner that can interest the reader or examiner and give them a clear idea of the subject matter written in the thesis. The introduction can be written during the course of the study, when the study data is being collected, or at the end of writing the thesis. It should be structured, brief, and concise. It should extend to no more than one or two pages. The introduction should start with statistics or key facts to draw the reader's attention to the topic. The importance of the research topic and its relevance in the current scientific world should be mentioned. The research question that was taken up in the thesis should be clearly mentioned in a simple way. The main job of the introduction is to tell readers why the researcher undertook the study. The introduction should clarify what the author's (researcher's) work adds on to the existing knowledge on the topic and touch upon the novelty of the research.

Essential Contents of Introduction

- Statement of general topic and background information.
- Definition of terms and scope of the research topic.
- Mention of current lacunae in information on the topic and the need for the study.
- Clear statement of the research question and hypothesis.

The sentences in the introduction that are picked up from other publications should be suitably superscripted with the number of the article that is cited in the References section. Mistakes commonly made while writing an introduction include—inability to state clearly the research question of the study, inclusion of review of literature, too long an introduction, and failure to define the need for the study.

THE AIMS AND OBJECTIVES

Every researcher should know what are the aims and objectives of the study before starting the study because an aimless study means a study without a foundation. A researcher without aims and objectives for his/her study is like a driver driving without a clear destination in mind. Not only should a researcher have aims and objectives, but these should be well-defined. Aims and objectives provide a clear direction and purpose for the study and help the researcher to stay focused and avoid getting off-track during the course of the study. Though aims and objectives sound similar and are interconnected, they are two distinct entities which serve different purposes.

Aims Section

These are general statements that describe the overall purpose of the research study. They are broad in scope and provide a general direction for the research. They are written in a general, abstract, and theoretical manner to depict the ultimate goal of the research study.

Example: To investigate the impact of sevoflurane administration on perioperative outcomes.

Objectives Section

These are specific, measurable, and achievable goals/endpoints that the researcher wants to accomplish within a specified time frame. These are statements that describe activities/tasks/steps that need to be carried out to achieve the aims of the research. They are narrower than aims in scope and provide specific details about how the research will be carried out. Unlike aims, objectives are concrete and operational. They are **s**pecific, **m**easurable, **a**chievable, **r**elevant, and **t**ime bound (SMART).

Example: Determining the impact of sevoflurane induction on emergence delirium.

Objectives can be *primary and secondary*. The primary objective is the most important endpoint and should reflect the research question. The additional endpoints which we want to study are termed as the secondary objectives.

Confusion between Aims and Objectives

Very few students and researchers understand the true meaning of "aims and objectives" and they often think that these terms are synonymous. However, it is pertinent to note that aims provide a broad context and final destination of the research, whereas objectives provide the small steps that the researcher must climb to reach the ultimate goal. Aims indicate what is to be achieved and objectives indicate how it is to be achieved. Objectives divide the aims into smaller parts. Well-defined aims and objectives ensure that the study remains relevant and meaningful, make the researcher stay focused on the research topic, guide the research design, help with effective allocation of resources, and assist in evaluating research by finding out whether the aim has been met and the research has reached its goals. They enhance communication and foster collaboration among the research team members.

How to Frame the Aims and Objectives?

They should be framed in such a way as to establish the scope, depth, and ultimate direction of the research. They can be devised based on the research question and after doing a good literature review. Action verbs such as "investigate", "evaluate", "compare", "find out", and "analyse" can be used while framing the aims and objectives.

Common mistakes found in the framed aims and objectives include too general/unclear aims and objectives with lack of focus, too narrow/specific aims and objectives, framing too many unrealistic objectives, no matching with the research hypothesis, nonfeasibility in terms of time, budget, and resources, and unethical objectives that can jeopardise the research participants' safety.

An Example of Well-framed Study Objectives Matching the Title

- *Title of the study:* Comparison of efficacy of ketamine and fentanyl for pain relief during burns dressing
- *Aim of the study:* Compare the effectiveness of analgesia provided by ketamine and fentanyl for dressing change in burns patients.
- *Primary objective:* To compare the percentage change in pre- and postprocedure pain score between patients receiving fentanyl or ketamine for dressing change in burns intensive care unit.
- *Secondary objectives:*
    - To compare patient satisfaction regarding pain relief by using Likert scale.
    - To compare the changes in haemodynamic response during procedure in these patients.
    - To compare the side effects of ketamine and fentanyl in these patients.

- *Conclusion (A well written conclusion which matches the objectives stated):* Both fentanyl and ketamine provided adequate analgesia during burns dressing, but fentanyl offered better analgesia than ketamine. Haemodynamic parameters such as heart rate, systolic and diastolic blood pressure were better controlled with fentanyl group during the procedures. Patient satisfaction for the analgesia provided was also better with fentanyl group.

What are Outcomes?

Outcomes are the measurable endpoints of objectives which are monitored during the study. The occurrence and absence of the outcomes indicate that the results have been achieved. The outcomes should originate and be in alignment with the objectives. The outcomes of the study need to be defined a priori and a standard validated method should be mentioned to measure them.

Examples of Objectives and Outcomes

- *Aim:* To determine the degree of hypotension of a new drug as compared to a standard induction agent.
- *Primary objective:* To evaluate the degree of hypotension after its administration and compare it with the effect of an agent in clinical use.
- *Primary outcome:* To determine whether a significant reduction in mean arterial pressure occurs with the new drug compared to a standard induction agent.
- *Secondary objective:* Recording other adverse effects of the drug.
- *Secondary outcome:* Recording of rash along the venous path; events such as cough after its administration.

REVIEW OF LITERATURE SECTION

It is a survey of published materials relevant to a particular area of research, for example, the topic of the dissertation. It provides a description summary of each published article related to the topic of research and critically evaluates the research work depicted in the article. Review of literature can help identify "gaps" in the literature and scientific knowledge related to the topic of research.

A well written review of literature provides the readers with background information necessary to understand the work of the researcher. It provides a thorough and critical outline of the intellectual developments in the field of research and resolves conflicts between differences in observations of different research studies. It can provide new perspectives on the previously published work related to the topic.

Search strategies for review of literature include using keywords, Medical Subject Headings (MeSH) terms, filters, publication type and date, databases on search, Boolean search strings, and exclusion criteria in search (*Example:* **Annexure 7**).

Review of literature should be done stepwise. The steps include:

- Identification of sources of literature
- Reading the sources
- Listing the sources
- Identifying gaps in existing scientific knowledge
- Writing the review of literature

Identification of Sources of Literature

- Primary
  - Articles published in peer reviewed journals
  - Preliminary reports/conference proceedings
- Secondary
  - Systematic reviews
  - Meta-analyses
- Tertiary
  - Books

Literature search can be done in two ways:

1. Library searching
2. Web-based methods using search engines and evidence-based databases.

Examples: Google/Google Scholar/Yahoo search engines and electronic databases such as PubMed, MeSH, Medline, CINAHL, Embase, etc.

Reading Sources of Literature

One should initially go through all articles' texts to get an idea of their general content. The next step would be to adopt a focused approach and read the abstract of each article followed by the introduction and conclusion part of the article. Each article of interest is next read in depth and critically especially in relation to the methodological approach, discussion, and general hypothesis.

Listing Sources of Literature

A list of the identified sources of literature can be made using reference tools such as Mendeley that can allow one to store the reference sources online and via a desktop application. Citation tools that are attached to these programs will help export citations in a chosen format later on, when writing and citing the references at the end of the dissertation.

Identification of Research Gaps

A gap means a lacuna or missing piece of information on the topic of research. It means that researchers have not yet touched upon this part and that this information has to be obtained by future research. The hypothesis related to the topic of current research should ideally help to fill the research gaps.

It should be written under subheadings related to the topic of dissertation.

Example: If the topic is "Assessment of airway changes during pregnancy with ultrasonography and clinical airway screening tests: a prospective observational study", the subheadings for the review of literature would be:

- Airway assessment in an adult
- Anatomical and physiological changes of pregnancy with focus on airway changes in pregnancy
- Basics of ultrasonography including technique and devices
- Sonographic measurements and assessment of airway.

Studies related to the topic of the thesis or published studies that are similar to the topic of the research are described in the review of literature. One can use third person phrases such as: "Dasgupta, et al. are of the view that...." or "the authors of a study concluded that". The studies selected for the review can be described in brief with respect to the aims, methodology, observation, and conclusion.

Example: In a study on five obese patients and seven morbidly obese adults, a submandibular sonographic examination performed in the supine position showed that the sonographic hyomental distance ratios in the difficult intubation group were in the 1–1.05 range and those in the easy intubation groups were in the 1.12–1.16 range, thus showing that the preoperative assessment of the hyomental distance ratio may predict difficult laryngoscopy resulting in difficult intubation.[23] Here, 23 stands for the citation number of the concerned reference article cited in the reference part. Studies can be quoted and described in series in this way in a chronological order depending on the year of published article, viz. 2019 study followed by 2020, 2021, and so on up to date. The most recently conducted studies should always be included. Newer articles, especially of previous 5 years, should be given preference. One can also start with the most recent article and go back chronologically.

Tips for Writing Review of Literature

- One should be selective while reviewing research and choose key papers related to the topic. It is not necessary that every piece of literature related to the topic should be reviewed. However, the review should be up to date and should not miss out on important, good quality articles that have robust study designs.

- Review of literature can include review of published original research articles and conference papers.
- One should write in simple language and use formal style of writing.
- Using strong or personal language is not advisable.
- The sentences should not be plagiarised, that means sentences should not be picked up verbatim from the source of literature and entered in the review of literature without superscripting them with the concerned reference.
- The sentences that refer to published literature should be superscripted with the concerned reference, viz. the number of the reference in the bibliography.
- It is easy to access articles from the web. However, one should select articles that appear authentic and are published in standard journals.
- A systematic record of all references should be kept while writing review of literature. These have to be mentioned later on in the bibliography/references section.

THE REFERENCES SECTION

We look further by standing on the shoulders of giants. This is the core of the ethical principle behind citation, and therefore they should be relevant and attribute the credit of primary discoveries/inventions appropriately. Scientifically, no research is done in isolation and citations, viz. references are what indicate the previously published work that we are referring to at various stages during our thesis. The sources of literature from which one takes sentences or ideas or information for the dissertation become the "References". These are to be written in an orderly fashion in the part of the dissertation known as References/Bibliography. These references are usually entered in Vancouver style in the text part of the manuscript (the reference number is superscripted in brackets next to relevant text) i.e., they should appear in the same consecutive numerical order as they appear in the final references section.

The correct punctuation marks should be used while writing references. "et al". can be used after 6 authors if the referred article has >6 authors.

Book references, web-based references, and journal references are to be written in a typical style.

Example of a Correctly Written Journal Article Reference

Jarvik JG, Maravilla KR, Haynor DR, Levitz M, Deyo RA. Rapid MR imaging versus plain radiography in patients with low back pain: initial results of a randomized study. Radiology. 1997;204:447-54.

Example of a Correctly Written Book Reference

Bajwa SJ, Kurdi MS. Endocrine surgery. In: Dinsmore J, Zoumprouli A, editors. Lee's Synopsis of Anaesthesia. 15th ed. Gurgaon: RELX India Pvt. Ltd; 2023. pp.643-62.

Example of a Correctly Written Web-based Reference

Cancer-Pain.Org [homepage on the Internet]. New York: Association of Cancer Online Resources, Inc; c2000-01 [updated 2002 May 16; cited 2002 Jul 9]. Available from: http://www.cancer-pain.org/.

Few Examples of Badly Written References

- *Assistant professor, department of anaesthesia and Intensive Care, Queen's Institute of Medical Sciences Hyderabad Telangana, MD DSPMBBS. Comparison of epidural Fentanyl and Buprenorphine as Adjuvants to Bupivacaine in Lower Abdominal Surgeries:*

A randomized clinical Study. J Med Sci Clin Res. 2016 Dec 23;04(12):14842-7.

- *Dept of Anaesthesia, Rajah Bhoj Medical College and Hospital, Chidambaram, Tamil Nadu, India, Sittaramane DS. A Comparative Study of the Effect of Fentanyl 25MCG with Bupivacaine 0.5% Verses Buprenorphine 60 MCG with Bupivacaine 0.5% in Spinal Anaesthesia for Elective Caeserean Section. J Med Sci Clin Res [Internet]. 2017 Nov 15 [cited 2022 Jan 21]; 5(11).*
- *Post Graduate, Department of Anaesthesiology, BEMS, Muppala DBM. Comparative Study of Epidural Injection of 0.5% Bupivacaine with Buprenorphine and 0.5% Bupivacaine with Fentanyl for Lowe Limb Surgeries. J Med Sci Clin Res [Internet]. 2020 Nov 20[cited 2022 Jan 22]; 08(11).*
- *Baird WLM, Reid AM. The neuromuscular blocking properties of a new steroid compound, pancuronium bromide. A pilot study in man. Br J Anaesth. 1967.39;775:80.*

Citation Management

Depending on the breadth and depth of the inquiry, the references may run into hundreds of documents. If not organised properly, referencing and making bibliography in the thesis often becomes a time consuming and stressful affair. Citation management software are tools which facilitate this process, and with some effort in organising, they can create the bibliography section at the click of a button, make it very easy to modify it several times and format it as per various citation styles. Some of the key features of this software are reference collection and organisation, automatic citation and bibliography generation, integration with word processors such as MS Word, Pages, etc., collaboration and sharing, and PDF annotation and note taking. Popular tools which serve this purpose include Zotero, Mendeley, EndNote, RefWorks, and BibTeX.

CONCLUSION

The initial parts of a dissertation, including the introduction and review of literature, should be written in a systematic and organised way by referring to literature related to the topic and by having a clear idea of the study. The title, aims and objectives, and abstract are important headings of a dissertation which should be brief, scientifically accurate and concise. These headings of the dissertation form the pillars on which the remaining part of the dissertation is built.

BIBLIOGRAPHY

1. Bajwa SJ, Sawhney C. Preparing manuscript: Scientific writing for publication. Indian J Anaesth. 2016;60(9):674-8.
2. Compilatio. How do you write a good introduction to a thesis or dissertation? [Online] Available from https://www.compilatio.net/en/blog/introduction-thesis [Last accessed July, 2025].
3. DISCOVERPHDS. Aims and Objectives-A guide for academic writing. [Online] Available from https://www.discoverphds.com/advice/doing/research-aims-and-objectives [Last accessed July, 2025].
4. Moss F. Titles, abstracts and authors. In: Hall MG (Ed). How to write a scientific paper, 3rd edition. Navarra: BMJ Publishing Group; 2003. pp. 42-50.
5. Scribber. How to write a thesis or dissertation introduction. [Online] Available from https://www.scribbr.com/dissertation/introduction-structure/ [Last accessed July, 2025].
6. Smith R. Introductions. In: Hall MG (Ed). How to write a scientific paper, 3rd edition. Navarra: BMJ Publishing Group; 2003. pp. 6-15.
7. Thomas R. Research aims and objectives: The dynamic duo for successful research. [Online] Available from https://www.enago.com/academy/research-aims-and-objectives/ [Last accessed July, 2025].
8. UNSW students. How to write a thesis introduction. [Online] Available from https://www.student.unsw.edu.au/introductions [Last accessed July, 2025].
9. Websites of scientific journals.

8

CHAPTER

Basic Statistical Tests

Prasad S

INTRODUCTION

Several questions can arise in researchers' minds at different stages of their research. The sections in this chapter are devised in such a way that undergraduate/postgraduate (UG/PG) students who are conducting research can get an answer to these queries. The first three sections deal with data and descriptive statistics, while the remaining deal with the pathway to inferential statistics.

Q1. I am confused that I have a lot of entries to be made, I have numbers such as age, duration of hospital stay, values of markers, Sequential Organ Failure Assessment (SOFA) score, Visual Analogue Scale (VAS) pain score, etc. on one hand, while classifications such as severity of disease (mild, moderate, and severe), outcome (survival or death), groups of people, etc. on the other hand. I wanted to know about these and how should I interpret them?

Ans: The answer for your query is explained in *Section 1* with suitable examples. This forms the basis for further chapters. As we all know, "*weight*" can be mentioned in kilograms or pounds, "*data*" are classified in this way.

Q2. I have got a clear idea about the various types of categorical data that are captured in research studies. But I wanted to know how to describe them during a presentation or thesis?

Ans: *Section 2* details the descriptive methods used for categorical data that are classified according to the researcher's wish or any predetermined methods. These are nothing but the illustration of measurements one makes while doing research. Both, the independent variables (risk factors/exposure) and the dependent variables (outcome) may take this function.

Q3. I have got a clear idea about the various types of numerical data that are captured in research studies. But I wanted to know how to describe them during a presentation or thesis?

Ans: *Section 3* details the descriptive methods used for quantitative data. The numerical data that are measured will be represented either separately for a group (e.g., age distribution of the study population), compared between the groups (e.g., age distribution of the males and females), or compared between them (e.g., age *vs.* weight).

Q4. Unlike categorical data that can be piled up into certain classes, the quantitative data has only numbers that range from a smaller value to larger ones. How will I know what measure should I take to represent these spectra of numbers? How will I know how dispersed are my data?

Ans: Universally, any happenings that are measured by values have this challenge and this is where summarisation of data is needed. The answers for these queries are given in *Section 3*.

Q5. On summarisation of data, we get a distribution and what am I going to do with that?

Ans: The distribution will remain as a blueprint for modeling or prediction of location of value, and one can make assumptions of which test to apply. The associations can also be inferred if two distributions are plotted simultaneously. The answers related to this are provided in *Section 4*.

Q6. I have collected data related to a diagnostic test(s) whose results are compared with another standard test. The results of the tests are compared between two consultants. How are they compared?

Ans: *Section 4* contains topics related to agreement and screening test that will be useful in understanding this concept.

Q7. In my study, I have to use a numerical value to predict the occurrence of an outcome. What should I do?

Ans: This will be an advancement of the screening test where receiver operating characteristic (ROC) curves are used. This has been explained with an example in *Section 4*.

Q8. With findings from my sample, how am I going to determine the values existing in the whole population? Will they be exactly the same or will there be any variations? I feel variations will be definitely present and how am I going to understand and address them?

Ans: *Section 5* elaborates the features of estimation and you will get the answers for this question.

Q9. Can I standardise my data and make this useful for comparison between studies of various geographical regions?

Ans: Z-distribution (Z-score) is the answer and is described in *Section 5*.

Q10. I have an important question. What is *p*-value?

Ans: This will be the purpose of conduction of research and is described in *Section 5*.

Q11. I have described the data and for inferential statistics, I do not know which tests to apply?

Ans: After knowing type of data, the predictions and derivation of *p*-value for giving the inference of the associations are portrayed in *Section 6*.

Q12. In my intervention, I have included "time" as one component in determining the occurrence of an event and how am I going to measure and interpret it?

Ans: Time-to-event studies are conducted rarely during UG/PG period owing to time constraints. The survival analysis and related tests are explained with examples in *Section 7*.

SECTION 1
DATA CLASSIFICATION AND EXAMPLES

Data consist of a group of observation of variables. A variable is any quantity that varies, for instance, we might gather basic clinical and demographic data on individuals suffering from a specific ailment wherein the patients' age, height, weight, and sex may be the factors of interest **(Flowchart 1)**.

Flowchart 1: Types of data.

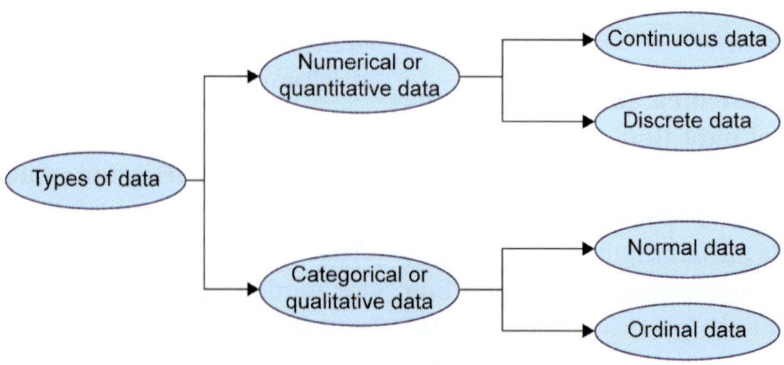

QUALITATIVE DATA

These occur when an individual can only be assigned to one of several unique categories for the variable.

Nominal

The categories just have names and are not arranged. Gender (male, female, transgender) and marital status (married, widower, single, etc.) are a few examples. There is no reason to think that being married in this situation is any better or worse than being alone. When a categorical variable has only two possible categories, it is binary or dichotomous. "Yes/no", "survivors/nonsurvivors", and "presence/absence of disease" are a few examples.

Ordinal

There is a hierarchy among the categories. Examples include the severity of discomfort (severe, moderate, mild, or none) and the illness staging systems (advanced, moderate, mild, or none).

QUANTITATIVE DATA

These occur when a numerical value is assigned to the variable.

Discrete

These arise when a variable accepts only whole numbers. These are frequently tallies of numbers of occurrences, such as the number of males who died with an illness or the total number of intubation attempts made in case of difficult intubation.

Continuous

A variable that can have any value within a given range is called a continuous variable, for example, weight, height, etc. The values of a continuous variable can include decimals (e.g., height measured in "cm" is meaningful even if it is in decimals such as 165.6, 165.7, 165.8, and 165.9, which then turns into a whole number "166.0" in the continuum). Furthermore, the quantification will be more appropriate. This means that if a 4-year old child normally weighs 20kg, and another child weighs only 10kg, then the second child's weight is exactly half that of the normal child.

Why should we know the types of variables?
We employ different statistical techniques for analysis depending on whether the data are numerical or categorical.

Special Note: Avoid documenting numerical data as categorical at the beginning (e.g., by noting each patient's age range rather than their actual age), as this can lead to the loss of vital information. Once obtained, numerical data can be easily converted to categorical data.

SECTION 2
DESCRIPTIVE METHODS FOR CATEGORICAL DATA

Categorical data can be described using two primary methods—*numerical and visual.* We can better comprehend the data distribution across many categories using both these approaches. In research, we generally get results that can be divided into two group or categories such as present or absent, male or female, improved or not, and normal or obtunded. The two outcome categories can often be designated as positive (+) and negative (–). If the primary category is observed, the outcome is positive; if the opposite category is detected, the outcome is negative.

On summarising the observations gathered about a group of people, it will be insufficient if we describe only the number of positives (number of observations, i.e., "x"). The number "x" provides very little information and only becomes significant when the group size, "n", is taken into account; in other words, the two figures, x and n, are frequently combined to create a statistic known as a *"proportion".*

$$p = x/n$$

Consider the following examples:

In one setting, number of cases of sepsis admitted in an intensive care unit (ICU) = 10, number of cases died within first 7 days = 5

The proportion here is 50% (or one out of every two).

In another setting, number of cases of sepsis admitted in ICU = 50 number of cases died within first 7 days = 5.

The proportion here is 10% (or one in every ten).

We need to understand that, in both these instances, the numerator is the same and this does not mean that both have same impact on the patient as it is clear that the proportion of patients who die is more in the first setting than in the later one.

EXPRESSING PROPORTIONS IN GRAPHS (VISUAL)

In a single glance, graphs provide significant information about the broad patterns of observations in a set of data. Consequently, it is usually easier to understand graphs than tables; as they are simple and self-explanatory.

Pie Charts

A *Pie chart* is made out of a circle with borders that represent the magnitude of the proportions for different categories. The differences in the sizes of various categories or subgroups (or wedges) as a breakdown of the total area are displayed in a pie chart. In the following figure, the various causes of sepsis are portrayed and all of them will total up to 100% **(Fig. 1)**.

Consider the following example where numerous causes of sepsis were studied and in such a scenario, a bar chart instead of a pie

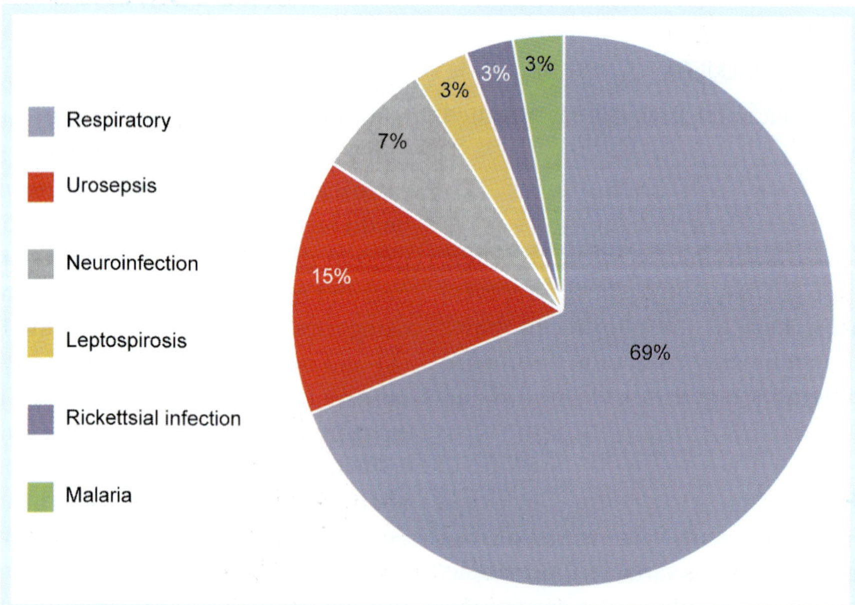

Fig. 1: Pie chart depicting the causes of sepsis.

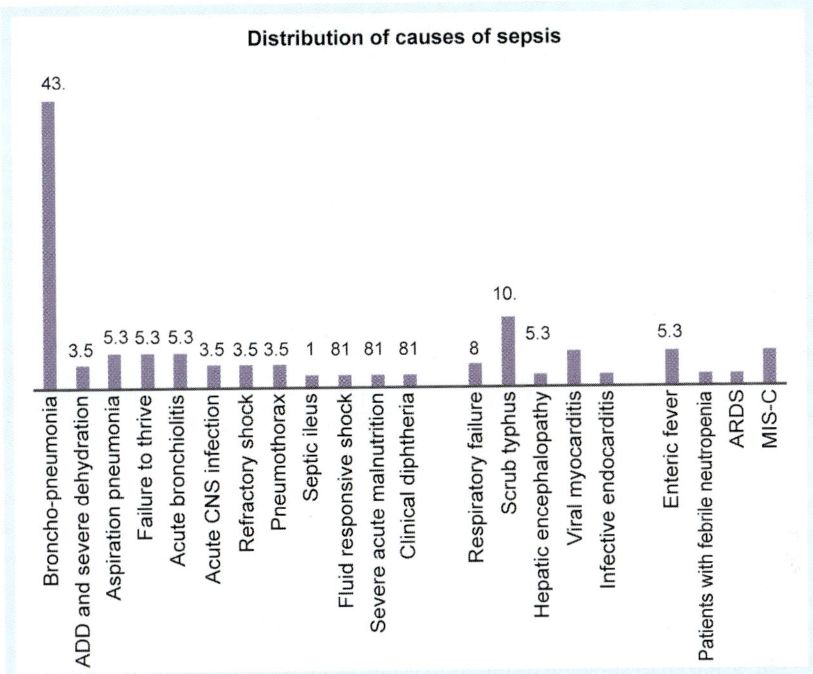

Fig. 2: Bar chart depicting the causes of sepsis. (ADD: acute diarrhoeal disease; ARDS: acute respiratory distress syndrome; CNS: central nervous system; MIS-C: miscellaneous)

chart will be easier to comprehend as the pie-chart becomes cluttered and difficult to interpret **(Fig. 2)**.

Bar Charts

Bar charts are also used to represent precise values or exact data values (expressed in proportions) as the bar heights are directly proportional to the values. It is advisable to use bar charts in place of pie-charts if the number of categories is more than three. Bar charts are excellent for displaying comparisons between several groups making it simple to determine which category has the highest, lowest, or comparable numbers. In **Figure 3**, it is clear that a higher percentage of non-survivors had rhonchi compared to survivors (27.7% vs. 11.7%) as compared against a higher percentage of survivors who presented with crepitations than non-survivors (55.9% vs. 41.7%). This makes the researcher investigate the causes that lead to these signs and arrive at a conclusion.

Line Graph

A *line graph* is similar to a bar chart which has "time" represented on the horizontal axis. Line graphs are best suited for situations where a single measure is monitored over an extended period of time. Since different "groups" represent consecutive time (hours or days or years), a line graph can be used to show how particular proportions vary over time. **Figure 4** represents the prevalence of obesity and severe obesity among adults aged 20 years or above that has significantly increased from 1999–2000 through 2017–2018.

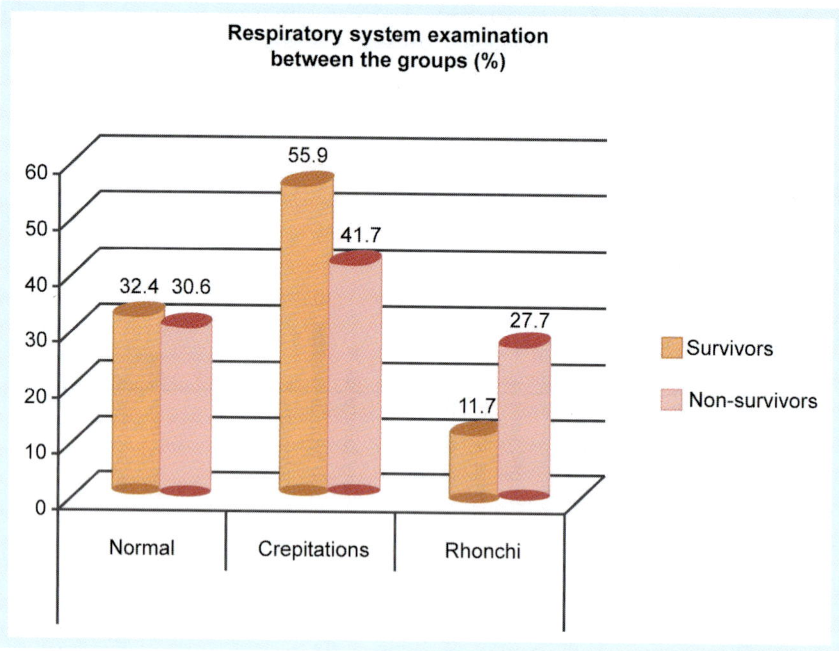

Fig. 3: Bar chart showing respiratory system examination findings in survivors and non-survivors.

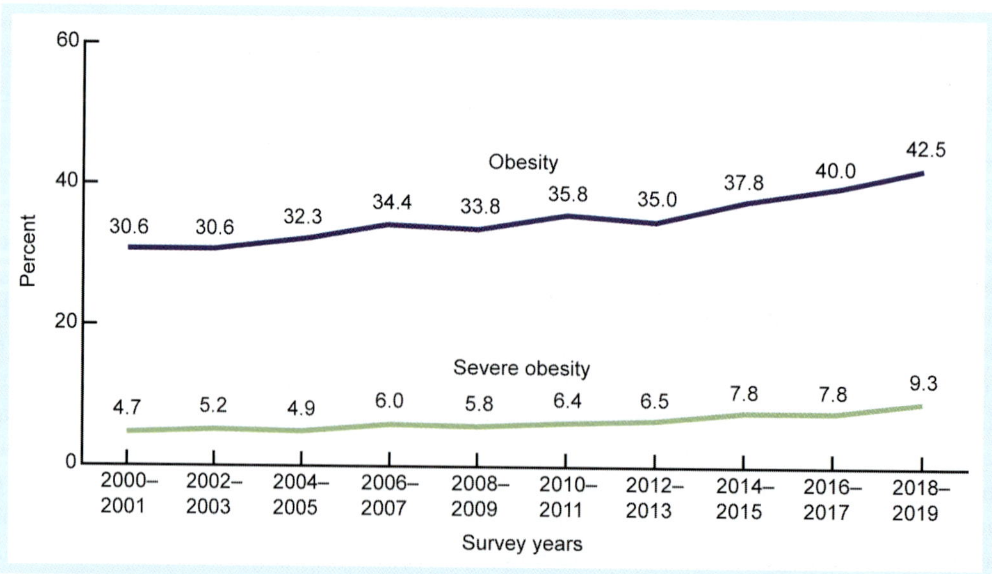

Fig. 4: Line graphs showing the prevalence of obesity and severe obesity among adults aged 20 years or above.

Line graphs can also be used to represent quantitative variables (e.g., change in heart rate, pain score over subsequent time intervals) which are described in the next *Section*.

RATES (NUMERICAL)

Rates, as opposed to proportions, are not static and they measure the frequency of events occurring during a specific time period. The term "rate" might be ambiguous because it can be used to indicate changes that occur after a specific amount of time or it can be used interchangeably with the term "proportion" to assess morbidity and mortality.

A proportion is a figure that falls between 0 and 100%, or between 0 and 1, but change rates might be higher than 100%.

$$\text{Change rate (\%)} = \frac{\text{new value} - \text{old value}}{\text{old value}} \times 100$$

According to a news article, the Centers for Disease Control (CDC) reported 35,238 new cases of Acquired Immunodeficiency Syndrome (AIDS) in 1989, up from 32,196 in 1988. On substitution of these values, the change rate was found to be 9.4% and this rate can be compared annually with the previous change rates so that one can evaluate the success of ongoing disease control programmes.

Similar rates for quantitative variables (e.g., change in heart rate, pain score between two time points) will be elaborated in the next *Section*. The morbidity and mortality rates can be displayed in a *crude* way (e.g., crude death rate) without considering age, gender, or race of a population. The variations between subgroups or disease categories are taken into account in *specific* rates (e.g., infant mortality rate, under-five mortality rate, etc.). Valid summary comparisons between two or more groups with dissimilar age distributions are achieved through the use of *adjusted* or *standardised* rates. (e.g., mortality comparisons between different countries or regions having varied age distribution). These are dealt with by epidemiologists.

RATIOS (NUMERICAL)

The formula for calculating a ratio is "a/b", where "a" and "b" are comparable quantities that are measured from various groups or under various conditions. Odds ratios (ORs) and relative risk (RR) are frequent ratios that we encounter in our research projects.

Relative Risk

In epidemiological investigations, "*RR*" is a notion for comparing two groups with respect to a specific undesired occurrence, such as sickness or death. In prospective research, it is traditionally expressed as the ratio of the incidence rates. The following examples give a good idea of understanding harmful or beneficial effects of some exposure:

$$\text{Relative risk} = \frac{\text{Incidence of cervical cancer in commercial sex workers}}{\text{Incidence of cervical cancer in females of general population}}$$

$$\text{Relative risk} = \frac{\text{Incidence of cervical cancer in human papilloma virus (HPV) vaccinated females}}{\text{Incidence of cervical cancer in females of general population}}$$

A RR is considered as a measure of association in cohort studies. A value above 1.0 denotes detrimental impacts, whereas a value below 1.0 denotes good outcomes. In the first example, the general population's female members typically live in standard settings, such as not being exposed to a certain risk factor, against which the group of commercial sex workers (*harmful* exposure) is measured. If RR = 2, the commercial sex workers are twice as likely to develop cancer of cervix compared to the females in the general population. In the second example, the females who are vaccinated are exposed to risk factor (*beneficial* exposure) that is mostly absent in the general female population. If RR = 0.5, it indicates that the females who got vaccinated with HPV vaccine have only half the risk of developing cervical cancer compared to the general female population.

Hazard Ratio

This is similar to RR, but is used in survival analysis (Section 7). *Hazard ratio* (HR) is calculated when the instantaneous risk of an event among the exposed group is compared against the instantaneous risk among the unexposed group at a specific time. A HR = 2 indicates that the exposed group is twice as likely to experience the event at any given time compared to the unexposed group.

Odds Ratio

In case-control studies, an OR is a statistical metric used to evaluate the relationship between an exposure and an outcome. It indicates the degree to which an occurrence is more (or less) likely to occur in one group than in another.

Odds: It is the probability that an event will occur divided by the probability that it will not, in simple terms, occurrence versus non-occurrence. For example, if odds of contracting flu are 2:1, it indicates a twofold increase in likelihood of acquiring it than the other possibility.

Exposure and odds: The OR typically compares the odds of an outcome (hip fracture) occurring in a group *exposed* to a certain factor (e.g., hormone replacement therapy or HRT) to the odds of the outcome occurring in a group with *no exposure* (e.g., no HRT).

Odds ratio and strength of association:

- An OR of *1* indicates *no association*. The odds of the outcome are the same in both the exposed and non-exposed groups.
- An OR >*1* suggests a *positive association*. The odds of the outcome are higher in the exposed group compared to the non-exposed group. The higher the OR, the stronger will be the association and the greater the likelihood of the outcome with exposure.
- An OR <*1* suggests a *negative association*. The odds of the outcome are lower in the exposed group compared to the non-exposed group. In other words, exposure might be protective against the outcome.

SECTION 3
DESCRIPTIVE METHODS FOR CONTINUOUS DATA

TABULAR AND GRAPHICAL METHODS

Scatter Plot

It shows the relationship between two continuous variables with one variable depicted on x-axis and another on y-axis. All data points are represented by dots that denote either the correlation, trends or patterns between the variables. In **Figure 5**, let us assume "height" and "weight" to be taken on x-axis and y-axis respectively. A positive correlation (Graph I) is indicated when as the height increases, the weight increases. Suppose that 'age' and 'insulin sensitivity' are considered on x-axis and y-axis, respectively, then as the "age" increases and the "insulin sensitivity" decreases (Graph II), a negative correlation is indicated. Graph III shows that there is no correlation between days of hospitalisation (x-axis) and improvements in Glasgow Coma Scale (GCS) score (y-axis).

Frequency Distribution

If the dataset is small, we can write the few numbers in ascending order, and the outcome will still be obvious. Hence, making a frequency

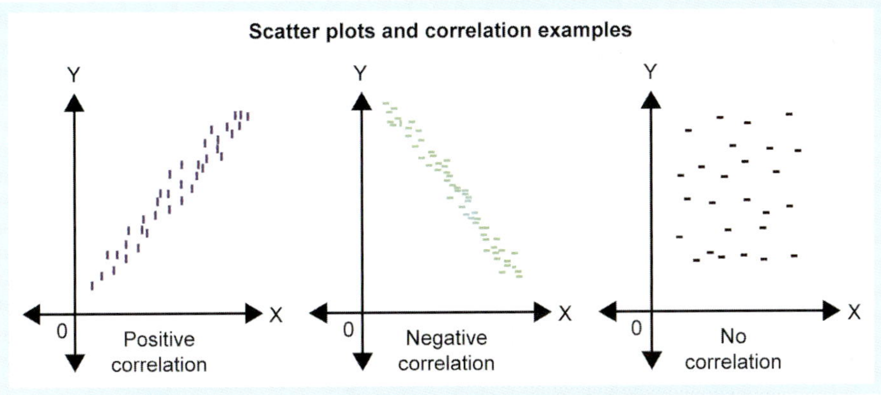

Fig. 5: Graphs I, II, and III showing scatter plots with correlation.

TABLE 1: Frequency distribution.

Age groups	*Frequency*	*Percentage*
<12 months	29	50.9
1–2 years	8	14.0
2–5 years	12	21.1
5–15 years	8	14.0
Total	57	100.0

table or frequency distribution will be a helpful tool for summarising somewhat bigger datasets.

Table 1 describes the frequency distribution age of one study population where the total number of study population is distributed across age groups, portraying the frequency (number of people) and the percentage of the overall population for each age group.

HISTOGRAM AND FREQUENCY POLYGON

A histogram, or frequency polygon, is a handy tool for showing a frequency table. A histogram shows the frequency or relative frequency in each interval on the vertical scale, with the value of the variable indicated at interval borders on the horizontal scale **(Fig. 6)**.

Cumulative Frequency Graph and Percentiles

A class of significant statistics known as percentiles or percentile scores is provided by the cumulative frequency graph. We would begin with the variable's smallest value and finish with its largest value on *x*-axis and the number of participants on the *y*-axis if we assume that we put our data in the order of magnitude. In the diagram below, the number of examinees and their scores obtained are depicted on "*x*-axis" and "*y*-axis", respectively. The dotted lines from both axes meet at a point (625,200), meaning that there are 200 examinees who obtained a score <625. This is where one has to know about percentiles, deciles, etc. **(Fig. 7)**.

The first percentile of an ordered collection of observations is the value of "x" at which 1% of the observations lie below it and 99% lie above it. The number that surpasses 90% of the values in the dataset and is only exceeded by 10% of them is known as the 90th percentile. The median is the term typically used to refer to the 50th percentile. *Deciles* are the values of "x" that, for an ordered set, divide it into ten equally sized groups (i.e., the 10th, 20th, 30th, and 90th percentiles).

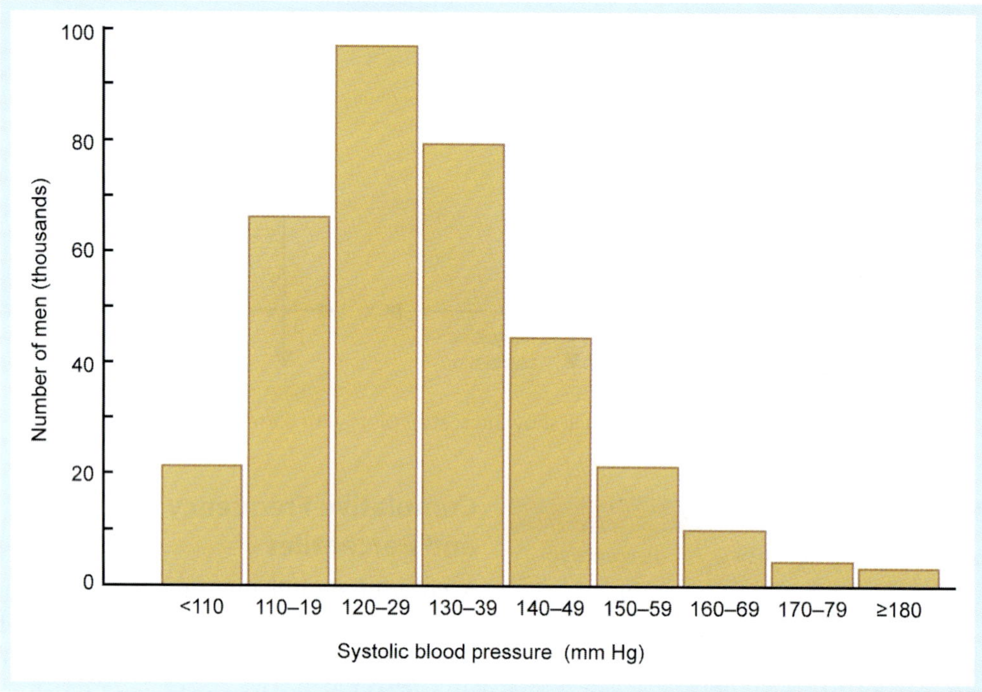

Fig. 6: Histogram or frequency polygon.

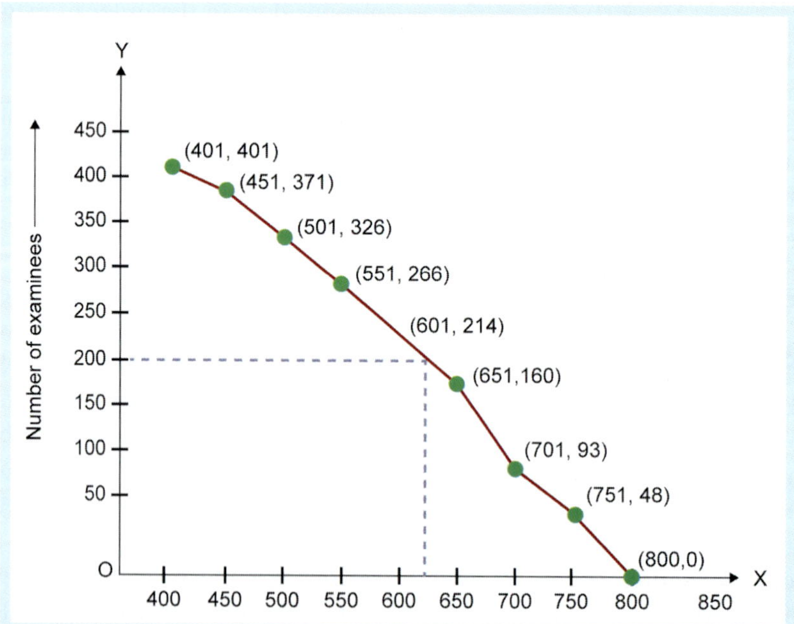

Fig. 7: Cumulative frequency graph.

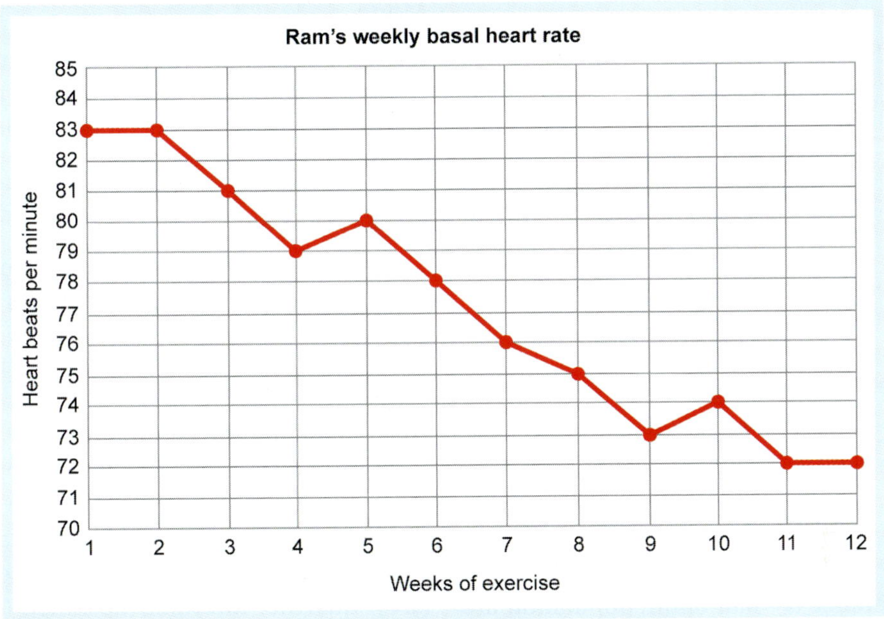

Fig. 8: Line graph.

Note: The National Eligibility cum Entrance Test (NEET) score, which is divided into several percentiles and arranged in an order (from lowest to highest), is the most typical example. The growth charts used in paediatrics for growth monitoring are another example.

Line Graph

A line graph, also known as a line chart or line plot, is a type of graph used to display information that changes over time. It consists of a series of data points connected by straight line segments on a grid.

The figure below demonstrates the change in heart rate over time (weeks of exercise). The time that we generally note is: preoperatively, on-table, 1-hour postoperative, 2-hour postoperative, etc. and the change in heart rate is noted. Multiple line graphs will be obtained if the heart rates of two or more groups are considered **(Fig. 8)**.

NUMERICAL METHODS

Measures of Central Tendency

It is also known as *central location or measures of centre* in a distribution of data. A summary measure endeavours to characterise an entire dataset by means of a "solitary value" that symbolises the midpoint or core of its distribution.

Mean, median, and mode are the measures.

Example: Out of 1,000 students, 12 are selected randomly. Their ages (in years) are given below and we are asked to calculate the measures of central tendency.

18, 18, 19, 19, 20, 20, 21, 22, 23, 23, 24, and 25

Mean

It is the mathematical average value of a set of data.

= Sum of the observations/Number of observations

= $\sum X_i/n$ (Where i = 1,2,3,.......12)

= 252/12 = 21

(i.e., Average age of the students is 21 years in the class)

Disadvantages: It is affected by extremes of values and is the preferred way to summarise if the data is normally distributed.

Median

It is the middle value in a distribution.

In order to find the median, all the observations (here, 12) have to be arranged in an *ascending order* as given below—

18, 18, 19, 19, 20, 20, 21, 22, 23, 23, 24, 25

Now,

Median = Middle value of the number of observations (n)
= {(n + 1)/2}th observation
= {(12 + 1)/2}th observation
= {13/2}th observation
= *6.5th observation from initial*
= Average value of 6th and 7th observation
= (20 + 21)/2 = 20.5

The inference is—half of the population are either younger than or equal to 20.5 years old, while the other half are older than or equal to 20.5 years old.

Median will be useful in summarising non-normally distributed data as it remains unaffected by the extremes of values(or outliers).

Mode

It is the most frequent number in a distribution.

To calculate, all the 12 observations are arranged in an ascending order as follows: 18,18, 19, 19, 20, 20, 21, 22, 23, 23, 24, and 25.

Mode = The most repeated observation is 18, 19, 20, and 23 (each repeated 2 times)

This distribution is thus multimodal. We generally use it for nominal variable in qualitative research.

Measures of Dispersion

Dispersion measures quantify the degree of variance or dispersion of values in a population or sample, and indicate how dispersed a set of data is. The examples are—standard deviation (SD), standard error (SE), range, coefficient of variation (CV), quartile, interquartile range (IQR), and percentile.

Mean Deviation (Table 2)

The mean deviation (also called the mean absolute deviation) is the mean of the absolute deviation of a set of data around the data's mean.

TABLE 2: Calculation of mean deviation.

Serial number	X_i	*Arbitrary value*	*(X_i—Arbitrary value)*	*I(X_i- Arbitrary value)I*
1	18		−2	2
2	18		−2	2
3	19		−1	1
4	19		−1	1
5	20	20	0	0
6	20		0	0
7	21		1	1
8	22		2	2
9	23		3	3
10	23		3	3
11	24		4	4
12	25		5	5
			Total	24

(X_i-values of individual variables)

For a sample size (n), the mean deviation is defined by:

$$\text{Mean deviation} = \frac{\Sigma |X_i - A|}{n}$$

Where, "A" is an arbitrary value.

Mean deviation = 24/12 = 2

It can also take the value "0". Despite the existence of an original deviation, it will lead us to believe incorrectly that the data points are concentrated in a single place.

Standard Deviation (Table 3)

It measures the degree of spread-out of the numbers.

- Its symbol is "σ" (the Greek letter sigma)
- It is just the square root of variance.

$$s = \sqrt{\frac{\sum_{i=1}^{n} (x_i - \bar{x})^2}{n - 1}}$$

$$= \sqrt{(62/11)} = \sqrt{(5.2)}$$

Standard deviation = 2.3

(s: standard deviation; n: sample; x_i: value of individual variable; $\bar{x}$: mean)

Variance

Variance, in statistics, is a measure that tells how spread out the data points are in a dataset relative to their mean (average). It is defined as the average of the squared differences from the mean. To calculate the variance, the following steps are applied:

1. Work out the mean
2. Subtract the mean from each number and square the result (the squared difference). Work out the average of those squared differences.

$$s^2 = \frac{\sum_{i=1}^{n} (x_i - \bar{x})^2}{n - 1}$$

(s: standard deviation; n: sample; x_i: value of individual variables; $\bar{x}$-mean)

TABLE 3: Calculation of standard deviation.

Sl. No.	*X_i*	*Mean*	*(X_i—Mean)*	*(X_i—Mean)^2*
1	18		−3	9
2	18		−3	9
3	19		−2	4
4	19		−2	4
5	20	21	−1	1
6	20		−1	1
7	21		0	0
8	22		1	1
9	23		2	4
10	23		2	4
11	24		3	9
12	25		4	16
			Total	62

(X_i-value of individual variable)

Mean deviation is measured in the same units as the original data. Variance is measured in squared units of the original data. Larger variance indicates that the data points are further from the mean on average.

Imagine a group of archers shooting arrows at a target. Variance helps to quantify how scattered the arrows are around the bull's eye (the mean). A high variance indicates that the arrows are spread out further from the centre, while a low variance suggests that they are clustered closer together. A higher variance suggests that the data points are further away from the mean on average. Conversely, a lower variance indicates that the data points are closer to the mean. In the medical field, it is used to assess the variability present in a test like biochemical test, optometric reading, etc.

Standard Error

The SE is a statistical term used to describe the *variability* of an estimate, particularly the estimate of a population mean based on a

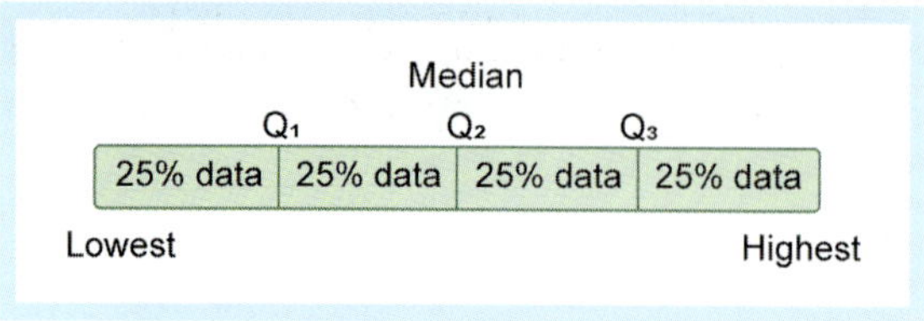

Fig. 9: Quartiles and data distribution. (Q_1: first quartile; Q_2: second quartile; Q_3: third quartile)

sample and reflects how much the sample mean will fluctuate if we draw different samples from the same population. A larger SE indicates that the sample mean is likely to vary more across different samples, and our estimate of the population mean is less precise.

Standard error = Standard deviation/√Sample size
= 2.3/√12 = 2.3/3.6 = 0.65

Quartile

In descriptive statistics, the quartiles of a ranked set of data values are the three points that divide the dataset into four equal groups, each group comprising a quarter of the data. A quartile is a type of quantile. The first quartile (Q1) is defined as the middle number between the smallest number and the median of the dataset. The second quartile (Q2) is the median of the data. The third quartile (Q3) is the middle value between the median and the highest value of the dataset **(Fig. 9)**.

For ith quartile = {i × (n+1)/4}th observation where i = 1, 2, 3

Second Quartile (Also Called Median or 50th Percentile)

= {2 × (n+1)/4}th observation
= {2 × (12+1)/4}th observation
= 6.5th observation
= Average of the 6th and 7th observation
= (20 + 21)/2 = 20.5

(i.e., 50% of students ages are either less or equal to the age of the 20.5 years)

Third Quartile (or 75th Percentile)

= {3 × (n+1)/4th observation
= {3 × (12+1)/4}th observation
= 3 × 13/4
= 9.75th observation
= 9th observation + 0.75 (difference between 10th and 9th observation)
= 23 + 0.75 × 0 = 23

(I.e., ¾th students' ages are either less or equal to the age of the 23 years.)

Interquartile Range

= 3rd quartile – 1st quartile
So, IQR = 23 – 19 = 4

Percentile

For ith percentile = {i × (n+1)/100}th observation
Where, "" = 1, 2, 3, ... 99

25th percentile:

= {25 × (n+1)/100}th observation
= {25 × (12+1)/100} = 3.25th observation
= 3rd observation + 0.25 (difference between 4th and 3rd observation)
= 19 + 0.25 × 0 = 19 = First quartile

Coefficient of Variation

The CV, also known as the relative standard deviation (RSD), is a statistical measure that describes the *relative spread* of a dataset compared to its mean. It expresses this spread as a *percentage*, making it easier to compare the variability of datasets with different units.

Unlike SD, which is measured in the same units as the data, CV focuses on the proportion of data spread around the mean. This allows for comparison between datasets with different units (e.g., weight in kilograms *vs.* height in centimetres).

Imagine there are two datasets:

1. *Dataset 1:* Weights of people (in kg) with a mean of 70 kg and a SD of 10 kg

2. *Dataset 2:* Heights of people (in cm) with a mean of 170 cm and a SD of 15 cm

Although SD is higher for heights (15 cm) compared to weights (10 kg), it is difficult to directly compare their spread due to different units.

The CV helps here:
- CV for weights = (10 kg/70 kg) × 100% = 14.29%
- CV for heights = (15 cm/170 cm) × 100% = 8.82%

Despite a higher SD, heights have a lower CV (8.82%) compared to weights (14.29%). This suggests that heights are proportionally less spread out relative to their mean as compared to weights of the population.

Box Plot

A graphical representation of a dataset that provides a visual sense of the position, distribution, degree, and direction of skewness is called a box plot. It also makes it possible to identify outliers. Box charts require a single horizontal axis, just as one-way scatter plots do. However, instead of charting each observation, they show an overview of the data. The components of a box plot are as follows:

From the 25th to the 75th percentiles, there is a central box. This box is split into two sections based on the dataset's median value. The distribution symmetry can be inferred from the relative diameters of the box's two sides. The dataset is roughly symmetric if they are roughly equal; if not, we can see the degree and direction of skewness.

The line segments that emerge from the box reach the nearby values in both directions. Little circles are used to symbolise each of the other data points outside this range; these are regarded as outliers or extreme observations that are not representative of the rest of the data.

In **Figure 10**, the severity of pancreatitis was assessed using Ranson's criteria and the patients

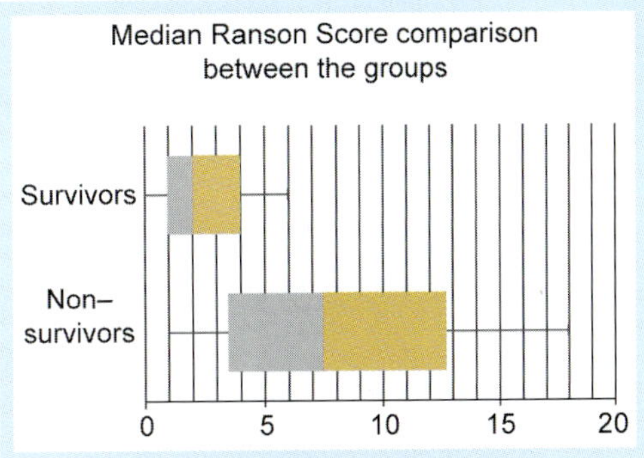

Fig. 10: Box plot showing median Ranson score between survivors and non-survivors.

were followed up throughout their hospital stay to study the association between Ranson's score and the mortality. The median Ranson's score for non-survivors is 7.5, whereas for survivors, it is 2. This indicates that higher Ranson's scores are associated with a higher risk of mortality in this study population. There are no outliers in the study population (no circles).

SECTION 4
PROBABILITY MODELS (NORMAL AND NON-NORMAL DISTRIBUTION) SCREENING, AGREEMENT, AND ROC CURVE

A probability model is a way to express mathematically the likelihood of various outcomes in a random phenomenon. It basically gives you a framework to understand the likelihood of certain things happening.

NORMAL DISTRIBUTION

A normal distribution, also known as the *Gaussian distribution* or *bell curve*, is a fundamental probability distribution in statistics. It is continuous, meaning that it represents the distribution of continuous data rather than

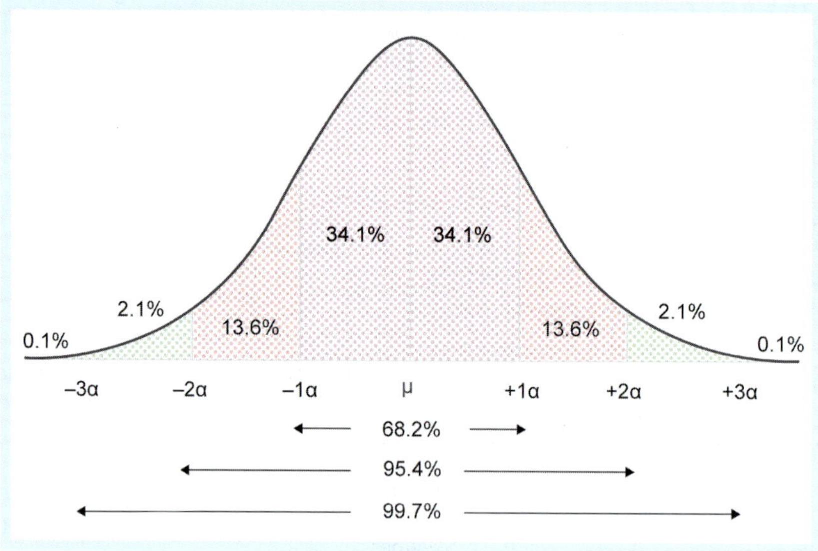

Fig. 11: The normal distribution showing bell-shaped curve.

discrete data. It is characterised by the following properties:

- *Symmetry:* The distribution is symmetric around its mean (μ), meaning the left and right sides of the curve are mirror images.
- *Mean, median, and mode:* In a normal distribution, the mean, median, and mode are all equal and located at the centre of the distribution.
- *Bell-shaped curve:* The curve of the distribution is bell-shaped, with most of the data points clustering around the mean, and fewer data points appearing as one moves further from the mean **(Fig. 11)**.

Empirical rule (68-95-99 rule):

- About 68.2% of the data falls within 1 SD (1σ) of the mean.
- About 95.4% falls within 2 SDs (2σ).
- About 99.7% falls within 3 SDs (3σ).

The reality is that a majority of the distribution that we get in our studies will not follow the normal distribution. If data is normally distributed, mean and SD can be taken as summary measures and if not, then median and IQR can be considered.

NON-NORMAL DISTRIBUTION

A non-normal distribution refers to any probability distribution that does not follow the characteristics of a normal distribution. In other words, it deviates from the symmetrical, bell-shaped curve exhibiting different characteristics such as skewness and kurtosis. Binomial and Poisson distributions are the most common occurrences.

Skewness

Positive Skew (Right-Skewed)

The distribution has a longer right tail. Most data points are concentrated on the left side, and the mean is greater than the median. An example of this is the duration of ICU stay among coronavirus disease (COVID)patients, most of whom died in the initial days, while a few sustained longer.

Negative Skew (Left-Skewed)

The distribution has a longer left tail. Most data points are concentrated on the right side, and the

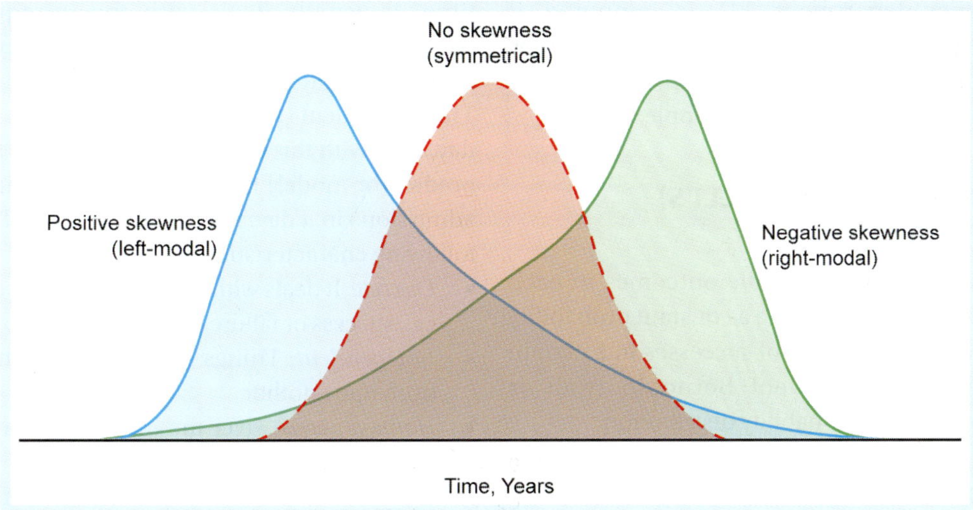

Fig. 12: Skewness of data

mean is less than the median. An example of this is the age at diagnosis of type 2 diabetes mellitus. Most patients will be diagnosed in the late 40s or early 50s; even the younger age groups may be diagnosed with the condition **(Fig. 12)**.

Kurtosis

Kurtosis is a measure that describes the shape of a distribution's tails in relation to its overall shape. A distribution can be sharply peaked with low kurtosis, and a distribution can have a lower peak with high kurtosis. Thus, kurtosis measures "tailedness," not "peakedness" **(Fig. 13)**.

Mesokurtosis

The extreme value feature of this distribution is similar to that of a normal distribution since its kurtosis is similar to that of a normal distribution. An example of this is the normally distributed weights of children in a classroom.

Leptokurtosis

With its long tails, or outliers, this distribution takes the shape of a curve. The majority of the

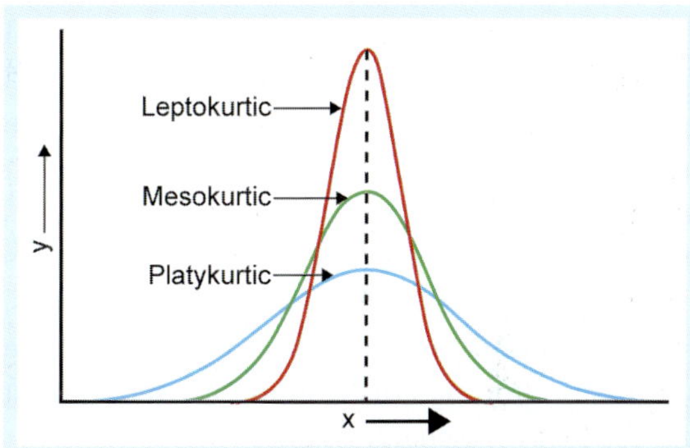

Fig. 13: Kurtosis of data.

data appears in a small ("skinny") vertical range due to the outliers, which extend the histogram graph's horizontal axis and give the distribution a leptokurtic appearance. An example of this is the average time taken for sedation for a group of patients for whom intravenous dexmedetomidine-ketamine were administered.

Platykurtosis

There are fewer outliers in the short tails of these distributions. For example, when the age distribution of patients getting admitted in an emergency department (ED) is computed, it will range from neonates to the elderly, thereby appearing flat with a small hump at the centre representing the middle-aged people.

BINOMIAL (BERNOULLI'S) DISTRIBUTION

There are only two possible outcomes in each trial: *success or failure*, with a constant probability of success. The number of successes in a certain number of independent Bernoulli trials is described by this probability distribution.

For example, a study is conducted to evaluate the success of autonomic neuroprosthesis; that means, whether noninvasive electrical spinal cord stimulation when applied to individuals with spinal cord injury can restore autonomic cardiovascular function (success) or not. A total of five such patients (five trials) are intervened with this autonomic neuroprosthesis, and the outcome is the presence or absence of restoration (success or failure). We can conclude that this method is effective if we get three successes (restoration of autonomic function); that means, we have to find the probability of getting three successes. Binomial distribution is used here. It has the following characteristics:

- *Fixed number of trials:* The number of trials in the experiment is fixed, and it is represented by the letter n.
- *Individual trials:* Every trial is conducted discreetly. There are two possible outcomes from any trial—success or failure.
- *Constant probability:* For every try, the chance of success, represented by p, stays constant.

Poisson Distribution

Given a known average rate of occurrence, it describes the likelihood that a given number of occurrences will occur in a particular length of time. It usually deals with the infrequently occurring events. For example, if the average number of patients getting admitted with Road Traffic Accident (RTA) in a health centre is 10 per day, then with this distribution one will be able to predict (or model) the probability of getting five admissions in a day. Poisson distribution has the following characteristics:

- *Discrete:* It deals with counting things or events, eg., success or failure, survival, or death.
- *Independent:* Things or events happen apart from one another.
- *Homogeneous:* Over the interval, the average rate of occurrence stays constant.
- *Rare events:* There is very little chance that two or more things will happen at the same time.

CHALLENGES WITH NON-NORMAL DISTRIBUTION

Kolmogorov–Smirnov Test

Before presenting data, we might not be knowing whether the distribution of our data is normal or non-normal. This test helps in differentiating normal and normally distributed data.

Log Transformation

If data is positively skewed, log transformation compresses the right tail and helps normalising it. It is also used when the variables are related multiplicatively rather than additively where log transformations linearise the relationship.

Squaring

If the data has heavy tails or is platykurtotic, squaring will be helpful in normalising the curve which can also be applied when negative values are present. After conversion, one has to apply Shapiro–Wilk test or visually inspect a Q-Q plot to know whether these transformations have resulted in normality or not.

AGREEMENT

Kappa agreement, also known as *Cohen's Kappa coefficient* (κ) or *inter-rater agreement,* is a statistical measure used to assess the degree of agreement between two or more raters or observers on a categorical scale. It is particularly useful in situations where the categories are nominal and the ratings are subjective. In cases of lower respiratory tract infections among adults, the degree to which two consultants taking rounds are able to detect the infiltrates in the X-ray film is variable (present or absent). For instance, the agreement for visualising infiltrates was 82.6% among inpatients (i.e., 82.6% of the times, both identified infiltrates among inpatients) and was only 55.2% for outpatients. Kappa takes into account the agreement occurring by chance and hence adjusts the observed agreement, providing a more reliable measure of *inter-rater reliability* compared to simple percent agreement. This means the above percentage of agreement will be analysed by adjusting for chances and represented in the form of "Kappa".

Kappa values range from –1 to +1, where a value of "0" indicates no agreement beyond chance; a value of 1 indicates perfect agreement; and negative values indicate less agreement than expected by chance. A commonly used guideline for interpreting kappa values is:

- *Less than 0.40:* Poor agreement
- *0.40–0.59:* Fair agreement
- *0.60–0.74:* Good agreement
- *0.75–0.90:* Very good agreement
- *More than 0.90:* Almost perfect agreement

Interobserver reliability: This includes not only the agreement in ratings but also the consistency in its application for rating criteria. For instance, this statistical method can be applied when the chest X-ray readings are repeated for two or three consecutive times and observations from three different consultants are recorded. Interobserver reliability can be measured using *intra-class correlation coefficients* (ICCs), which are useful when dealing with continuous data or multiple raters and this provides both, the frequency of agreement as well as the consistency in the application of rating criteria.

Screening

Any medical test used to determine a population's or a subgroup's likelihood of having a specific disease is referred to as a screening test. Its main objective is to identify possible illnesses or problems early. This can help with early intervention and treatment, which may improve results. Although screening tests are not diagnostic in nature, they are meant to identify a portion of the population that needs more in-depth testing to ascertain whether the disease is present or not.

In screening, a new test is compared with a "Gold Standard" in order to derive the sensitivity, specificity, positive predictive value (PPV) and negative predictive value (NPV). Specificity measures the percentage of true negatives—those who are accurately diagnosed as not having the disease—while sensitivity measures the percentage of true positives, or those who are correctly recognised as having the condition. These metrics aid in comprehending the reliability and accuracy of the screening test in differentiating between those who have the illness and those who do not.

In **Figure 14A**, the formulae to calculate the sensitivity, specificity, positive-predictive value (PPV), and negative predictive value (NPV) are given. In **Figure 14B**, the meanings of true positive, false positive, false negative, and true positive are provided so that visual clarity about the concepts can be obtained. A, B, C, D are the values entered in the four boxes of **Figure 14**A. A denotes value in Row 1 Column 1, B denotes value in Row 1 Column 2, C denotes value in Row 2 Column 1, D denotes value in Row 2 Column 2.

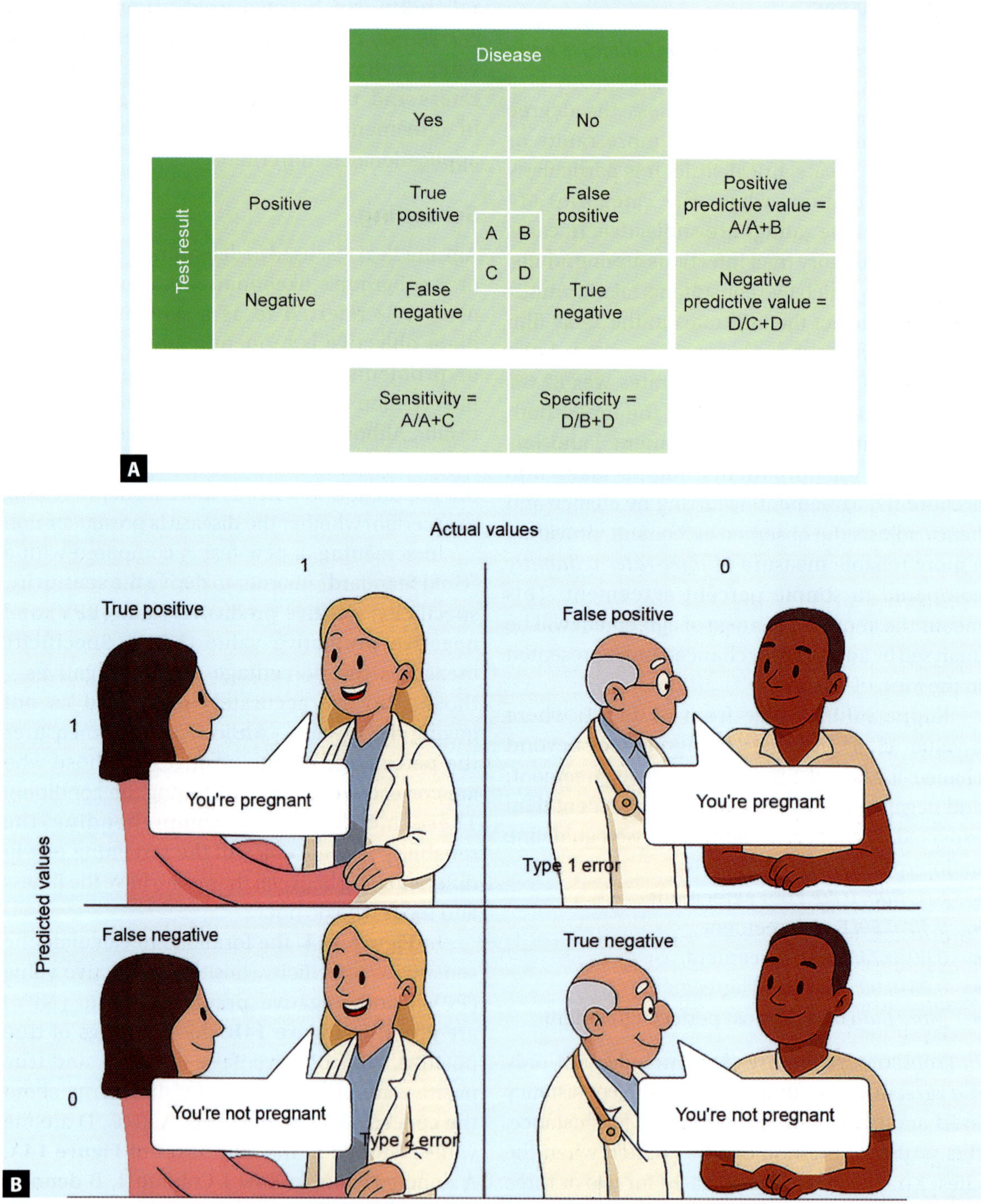

Figs. 14A and B: (A) Sensitivity, specificity, positive-predictive value, and negative-predictive value. (B) True positive, true negative, false positive, and false negative. (A, B, C, D represent values in each box as mentioned above in the text).

TABLE 4: Example of a screening test.

	Disease (+)	*Disease (–)*
Test +	450 (A)	150 (B)
Test	50 (C)	350 (D)

[A: true positive (TP); B: false positive; C: false negative; D: true negative (TN)]

Let us have a look at the following example and get the concepts clear. An intradermal test for newly developed filarial antigen was claimed to be effective in finding out the microfilarial carriers by the inventors. Out of the 1,000 persons injected intradermally with the antigen, the test was positive in 600 persons of whom 450 persons were really having the microfilaria in their peripheral blood. But the test was negative in 50 persons who were also having microfilaria in their peripheral blood. We shall now find out the parameters of this screening test **(Table 4)**.

Sensitivity = $A/A + C \times 100$

= True positive (a)/Total disease positive (a + c) × 100

= $450/500 \times 100 = 90\%$. A high sensitivity indicates the importance of early detection and avoidance of false negatives so that all diagnosed can be treated early.

Specificity = $D/B + D \times 100$

= True negative (d)/Total disease negative (b + d) × 100

= $350/500 \times 100 = 70\%$. A high specificity is important for avoiding false positives and preventing unnecessary interventions.

Positive predictive value (PPV) = $A/A + B \times 100$

= TP (a)/Total test positive (a + b)

= $450/600 \times 100 = 75\%$. A high PPV is required for making accurate diagnosis with a test and in guidance of treatment decisions.

Negative predictive value (NPV) = $D/C + D \times 100$

= TN (d)/Total test negative (c + d) × 100

= $350/400 \times 100 = 87.5\%$. A high NPV is required for reassuring patients and avoidance of unnecessary anxiety after the test results.

RECEIVER OPERATING CHARACTERISTIC CURVE

A ROC curve is a graphical plot that illustrates the diagnostic ability of a binary classifier model. It is used to evaluate the performance of a classification model by plotting the true positive rate (sensitivity) against the false positive rate (1 – specificity) at various threshold settings. Each point on the ROC curve represents a sensitivity/specificity pair corresponding to a particular decision threshold. The area under the ROC curve (AUC) is a measure of the model's performance, with a higher AUC indicating better classification performance.

For instance, a researcher wants to find the role of measuring the Q-SOFA score (quantitative variable) in predicting the prognosis (survival or death, a qualitative variable) of patients diagnosed with sepsis in the ED. ROC curve analysis was performed that was shown in **Figure 15** and **Table 5**.

Maximum sensitivity (96.0%) and specificity (86.7%) were found for the Q-SOFA score = 2.5. This curve was constructed for each value of Q-SOFA score that was observed among the sample of subjects. This value 2.5 bifurcated the groups into two, one was patients with Q-SOFA <2.5 and the other with Q-SOFA >2.5. On the other hand, the outcome would be survival or nonsurvival and hence we got a 2 × 2 contingency table from where the sensitivity and specificity were derived. ROC curve was thus constructed with each value of the input variable (Q-SOFA score), deriving the outcome (survival or not), eliciting the sensitivity and specificity and thereby developing this model. The AUC here is 0.925 or 92.5% meaning that the model is able to correctly distinguish between the survival and nonsurvival on taking Q-SOFA cut-off score = 2.5, 92.5% of the time. The confidence interval (CI) (95%) will be dealt with in the next *Section.*

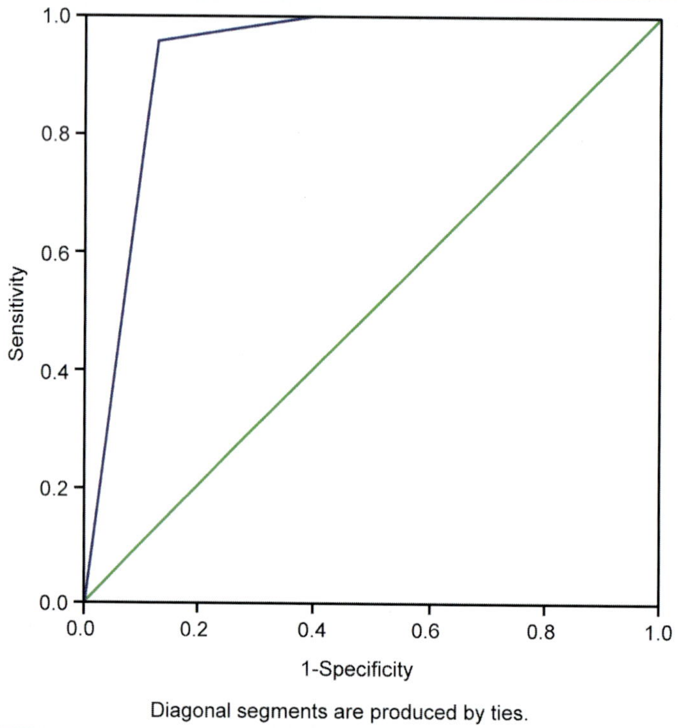

Fig. 15: ROC curve. (ROC: receiver operating characteristic)

TABLE 5: ROC curve analysis.

Area under the curve	Standard error	p-value	Asymptomatic 95% confidence interval	
			Lower bound	Upper bound
0.925	0.023	<0.001	0.880	0.970

(ROC: receiver operating characteristic)

SECTION 5 ESTIMATION OF PARAMETERS AND CORE CONCEPTS

(Sampling distribution, variance, SE of mean, CIs, estimation of proportions, Z-score, tests of significance, *p*-value)

ESTIMATION

After collection of data from a *sample*, any researcher would derive inferences about the *population*. It would be either value of some parameter (for example, success rate of newly developed vaccine) or comparison of parameters between two subpopulations using statistical tests of significance (for example, to know whether incidence of myocardial infarction is higher in postmenopausal women or elderly men). Estimation is nothing but a "best guess" as we use results from a sample *statistic* to guess about the population's *parameter*. Here, we should know that there exists a degree of uncertainty (or error)

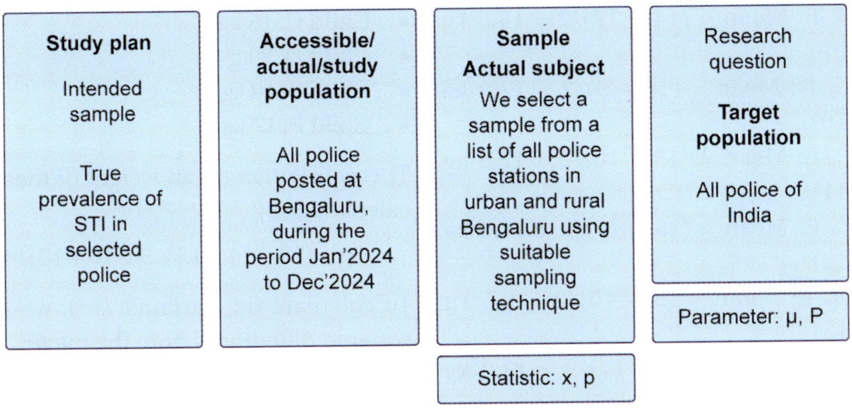

Fig. 16: Understanding study populations: From sample to target. (STI: sexually transmitted infection)

and that it may lie within a range of some nearby values (confidence limits).

A parameter is a numerical characteristic of a population; the population proportion "P" and mean "μ" are two examples of it. A statistic is the equivalent number derived from a sample. Sample mean "x" and sample proportion "p" are two examples of statistics (an example given in below diagram). We can make deductions or conclusions about population parameters with the aid of statistics. The value of a statistic (such as the sample mean "x") is known and fixed once a sample has been taken; if we take a different sample, we will almost certainly get a different numerical value for the same statistic. Within the context of repeated sampling, a statistic is viewed as a variable that varies in value across samples **(Fig. 16)**.

SAMPLING DISTRIBUTION

A statistical sampling distribution is the set of values for a given statistic that are derived from multiple identically sized samples taken from the same population. For instance, the weights of the children admitted in a paediatric intensive care unit (PICU) are as follows:

- *Child A:* 19 kg
- *Child B:* 14 kg
- *Child C:* 15 kg
- *Child D:* 9 kg
- *Child E:* 10 kg
- *Child F:* 17 kg

The *population* mean weight of these children is calculated as:

$$\mu = (19+14+15+9+10+17)/6 = 14 \text{ kg}$$

To illustrate the sampling distribution of the sample mean, we will take all possible samples of size "2" and calculate the mean of each sample.

Here are the possible samples and their means:

- Sample A, B: Mean = (19 + 14)/2 = 16.5 kg (Sample-1)
- Sample A, C: Mean = (19 + 15)/2 = 17.0 kg (Sample-2)
- Sample A, D: Mean = (19 + 9)/2 = 14.0 kg (Sample-3)
- Sample A, E: Mean = (19 + 10)/2 = 14.5 kg (Sample-4)
- Sample A, F: Mean = (19 + 17)/2 = 18.0 kg (Sample-5)
- Sample B, C: Mean = (14 + 15)/2 = 14.5 kg (Sample-6)
- Sample B, D: Mean = (14 + 9)/2 = 11.5 kg (Sample-7)
- Sample B, E: Mean = (14 + 10)/2 = 12.0 kg (Sample-8)

- Sample B, F: Mean = (14 + 17)/2 = 15.5 kg (Sample-9)
- Sample C, D: Mean = (15 + 9)/2 = 12.0 kg (Sample-10)
- Sample C, E: Mean = (15 + 10)/2 = 12.5 kg (Sample-11)
- Sample C, F: Mean = (15 + 17)/2 = 16.0 kg (Sample-12)
- Sample D, E: Mean = (9 + 10)/2 = 9.5 kg (Sample-13)
- Sample D, F: Mean = (9 + 17)/2 = 13.0 kg (Sample-14)
- Sample E, F: Mean = (10 + 17)/2 = 13.5 kg (Sample-15)

These sample means form the sampling distribution of the sample mean. The mean of all these sample means is:

$\bar{\mu}$ = (16.5 + 17.0 + 14.0 + 14.5 + 18.0 + 14.5 + 11.5 + 12.0 + 15.5 + 12.0 + 12.5 + 16.0 + 9.5 + 13.0 + 13.5)/15 = 14 kg

This example shows that the mean of the sampling distribution of the sample mean is equal to the population mean, which is a key property of the sampling distribution. This concept is crucial in statistics as it helps in understanding the variability of sample means and making inferences about the population from which the samples are drawn.

VARIANCE

A measure of dispersion or spread of a set of values is called variance. It measures the average distance between each value of the dataset and the mean value of the dataset. The average of the squared deviations from the mean is used to compute variance.

In continuation of the example quoted above, the weights of the children admitted in the PICU are:

- Child A: 19 kg
- Child B: 14 kg
- Child C: 15 kg
- Child D: 9 kg
- Child E: 10 kg
- Child F: 17 kg

The *population* mean weight of these children is calculated as:

$$\mu = (19 + 14 + 15 + 9 + 10 + 17)/6 = 14 \text{ kg}$$

To calculate the variance (σ^2), we first find the squared differences from the mean:

$(19 - 14)^2 = 25$
$(14 - 14)^2 = 0$
$(15 - 14)^2 = 1$
$(9 - 14)^2 = 25$
$(10 - 14)^2 = 16$
$(17 - 14)^2 = 9$

Then, we calculate the average of these squared differences:

$$\sigma^2 = 25 + 0 + 1 + 25 + 16 + 96 = 766 = 12.67 \text{ kg}^2$$

So, the variance of the children's weights is approximately 12.67 kg². If the weights of the children are more widespread, we will obtain a higher variance value which can be comprehended by from **Figure 17**.

STANDARD ERROR OF THE MEAN

The variability of a statistic from sample to sample is measured by the SE. It is a calculation of the sampling distribution's SD for a given statistic. It gives insights into how precisely the sample statistic estimates the population parameter.

First, recall the sample means we calculated for all possible samples (15 samples) of size two: 16.5, 17.0, 14.0, 14.5, 18.0, 14.5, 11.5, 12.0, 15.5, 12.0, 12.5, 16.0, 9.5, 13.0, and 13.5.

The mean of these sample means ($\bar{\mu}$) is 14 pounds, and the variance of these sample means (σ_x^2) is:

$$\sigma_x^2 = [(16.5 - 14)^2 + (17.0 - 14)^2 + \cdots + (13.5 - 14)^2]/(15 - 1) = 3.11 \text{ kg}^2$$

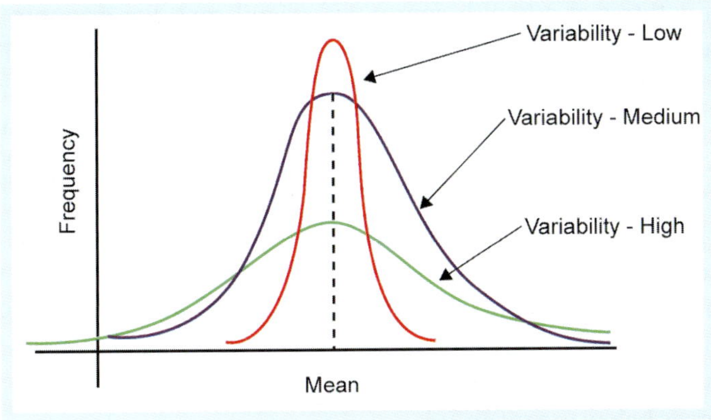

Fig. 17: Variance of data.

The standard error of the mean (SEM) is the square root of the variance of the sample means:

$$\text{SEM} = \sqrt{\sigma_x^2} = \sqrt{3.11} = 1.76 \text{ kg}$$

So, the SEM for the children's weights is approximately 1.76 kg.

CONFIDENCE INTERVAL OF MEAN

Given a specific degree of confidence, the range of values that comprise the true population mean is known as the CI of the mean. It can be calculated with the formula:

$$\text{CI} = \bar{x} \pm (Z \times s/\sqrt{n})$$

Where,

$\bar{x}$ is the sample mean

Z is the Z-score corresponding to the desired confidence level (i.e., 1.96 for a 95% confidence level)

s is the sample SD

n is the sample size

Hence, CI provides the estimate of the range of values within which the true population mean is going to lie. The width of the confidence estimate describes the precision of the estimate meaning, the more narrower the estimate the more precise the estimate is.

For example, in a sample size of 40 men, the average value of total cholesterol was 175 mmol/L with a SD of 20 mmol/L and with the above formula, the CI at 95% would be:

$$\begin{aligned}\text{CI} &= 175 \pm (1.96 \times 20/\sqrt{40}) \\ &= 175 \pm 6.20\end{aligned}$$

Hence, the 95% CI for the population's (overall men's) total cholesterol mean value as calculated from this sample would be lying between 168.8 and 181.2 cm.

Z-SCORE

A Z-score (standard score) is a measure that describes the position of a raw score (a measured value from sample) in terms of its distance from the mean, measured in units of SD. Any values or scores can be standardised using "z-score" so that they can be compared among various distributions. The Z-score is calculated using the formula:

$$Z = \frac{X - \mu}{\sigma}$$

Where,

X is the raw score

μ is the mean of the distribution

σ is the SD of the distribution

Suppose that in a sample of patients with alcoholic liver disease, one subject (Mr. A) had a serum glutamic-oxaloacetic transaminase (SGOT) value of 650 IU/L estimated using UV-Kinetic method. The mean value of SGOT for the whole sample of patients at a health centre was 500 IU/L, and the SD is 100 IU/L.

To calculate Mr. A's Z-score, we use the formula:

$$Z = 650 - 500/100$$
$$Z = 1.5$$

So, Mr. A's Z-score is 1.5. This means Mr. A's score is 1.5 SDs above the mean.

A Z-score of 0 indicates that the score is exactly at the mean. A positive Z-score indicates that the score is above the mean. A negative Z-score indicates that the score is below the mean.

In this example, Mr. A's Z-score of 1.5 indicates that his score is 1.5 SDs above the average score. This standardisation allows for comparison across different tests or distributions (example: SGOT computed by using other methods like spectrophotometric or coupled enzyme assays, immunological methods, etc.) as it provides a measure of how far a score is from the mean in a standardised way.

Applications of Z-Scores

- *Detection of outlier:* It is used to identify outliers in a dataset. Data points with Z-scores that are significantly different from 0 (e.g., greater than 3 or less than –3) are often considered outliers. For instance, if the Z-score for weight-for-age of a child is lying between -2 and -3, the child is classified as underweight. Furthermore, if the Z-score < –3, it denotes the child is severely underweight than others in its peer group.
- *Normal distribution:* Z-scores are used to standardise data to a normal distribution with a mean of 0 and a SD of 1. This standardisation allows for easier comparison and analysis of data across different datasets.
- *Hypothesis testing:* In hypothesis testing, Z-scores are used to determine the significance of results. A data point with a Z-score above a certain threshold (e.g., 1.96 for a 95% confidence level) is considered statistically significant. For example, a study was done to find mean systolic blood pressure (SBP) after intervening with an antihypertensive drug. A mean value that falls outside (Z-score <–2), indicates that the drug is effective in lowering the SBP.
- *Confidence intervals:* Z-scores are used to calculate CIs, which are used to estimate the range of values that a population parameter can take. This has been described earlier in this chapter.

ESTIMATION OF PROPORTION

Let us start with an example. A postgraduate student aimed to study 300 COVID positive cases and the purpose was to find those with oxygen saturation <90%. At the end of the study, he found 40 cases with peripheral oxygen saturation (SpO_2) <90%. With this available information, the calculated sample proportion would be:

$$p = 300/40$$
$$= 0.133$$

Similar to finding CI of mean, CI for the proportion can be found using the formula:

$$= p \pm Z \times \sqrt{p(1-p)/n}$$
$$= 0.133 \pm 1.96 \times \sqrt{0.133(1-0.133)/300} \quad (\text{Z-value} = 1.96)$$
$$= 0.133 \pm 0.038$$

The 95% CI for the true proportion of COVID cases with lower saturation (SpO_2 <90%) was (0.095, 0.171). This means that we are 95% confident that the true proportion of COVID cases with lower saturation (SpO_2 <90%) lay between 9.5 and 17.1%.

TESTS OF SIGNIFICANCE

A test of significance, also known as hypothesis testing, is a statistical method used to determine whether a hypothesis about a population parameter is true. It involves making an assumption about the population parameter

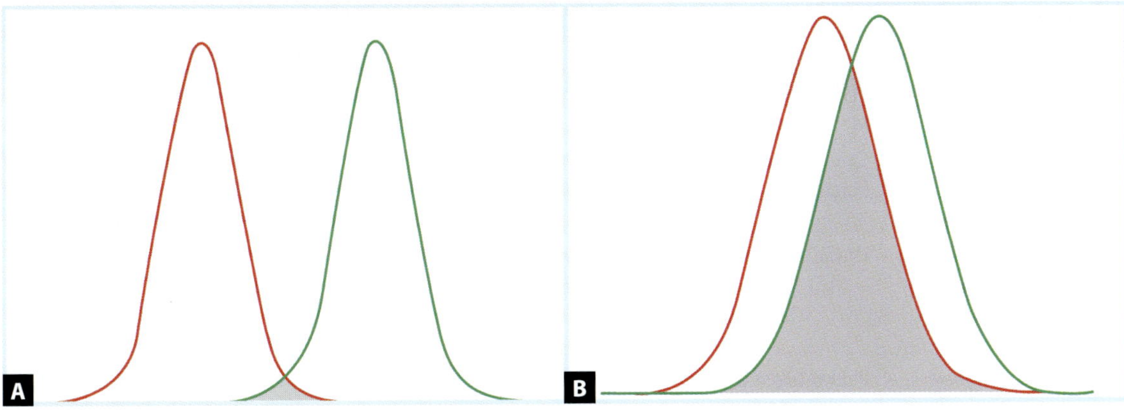

Fig. 18A and B: Null hypothesis association.

(the null hypothesis, H0) and then using sample data to determine whether there is enough evidence to reject this assumption in favour of an alternative hypothesis (H1). A study aimed to assess the existence of linear relationship between homocysteine levels and the myocardial ischaemia. Here, the null hypothesis would be non-existence of relationship (or association), while the alternate hypothesis would be presence of a significant relationship (or association) between homocysteine levels and myocardial ischaemia **(Figs. 18A and B)**. All the tests are described with examples in the next *Section*.

p-VALUE

It is the probability of getting the results of the study more extreme—if the null hypothesis is true. Rather than the sample, the null hypothesis is related to the population of interest. We conclude that there is insufficient data to reject the null hypothesis if the *p*-value is ≥0.05. We state that the data are not significant (significantly associated) at the 5% level and do not reject the null hypothesis. This merely indicates that there is *insufficient evidence* to rule out the null hypothesis and *not that, it is true*. Conversely, we believe that there is *enough evidence* to reject the null hypothesis if the *p*-value is <0.05 since there is a minimal possibility that the results would occur if the null hypothesis was true. We declare that the data are significant at the 5% level and *reject* the null hypothesis.

In **Figure 18A**, null hypothesis will be accepted because there is no association between two distributions (abnormal homocysteine levels and myocardial infarction) as the congruence between them is very less (or getting more extreme results) with the evidences that are available. The null hypothesis will be rejected and alternative hypothesis will be accepted **(Fig. 18B)** as there is a significant association between both the distributions as far as the evidences reveal.

SECTION 6
STATISTICAL TESTS OF SIGNIFICANCE

Table 6 outlines how to choose appropriate *summary measures* and *statistical tests* based on the *type of data distribution* (normal, non-normal, or binomial) and the *study design* (number and type of groups compared).

EXAMPLE-1: ONE SAMPLE T-TEST

A pharmaceutical company claims that its new drug can lower the blood pressure by 10 mm Hg (*quantitative—continuous variable*) within 1 week. To test the effectiveness of this drug, a clinical trial was conducted wherein 75 patients

TABLE 6: Common statistical tests based on type of data distribution and study design.

Measurements Groups	*Normal or Gaussian distribution*	*Non-normal distribution*	*Binomial (two outcomes)*
One group	Mean, standard deviation	Median, interquartile range	Proportion
Comparison of one group to a hypothetical value	One sample t-test (Example-1)	Wilcoxon Rank–Sum test (Example-2)	Pearson's Chi-square test (Example-3)
Comparison of two unpaired groups	Unpaired t-test (Example-4)	Mann–Whitney U test (Example-5)	Fisher's exact Chi- square test (Pearson's Chi-square test for larger groups) (Example-6)
Comparison of two paired groups	Paired t-test (Example-7)	Wilcoxon test (Example-8)	McNemar's test (Example-9)
Compare three or more unmatched groups	One-way ANOVA (Example-10)	Kruskal–Wallis ANOVA test (Example-11)	Pearson's Chi-square test (Example-12)
Compare three or more matched groups	Repeated measures ANOVA (Example-13)	Friedman test (Example-14)	Cochrane-Q (Example-15)
Quantitative association of two variables	Pearson's correlation (Example-16)	Spearman's correlation (Example-17)	—
Predict value from another measured variable	Simple linear regression or nonlinear regression (Example-18)	Nonparametric regression (Example-19)	Simple logistic regression (Example-20)
Predict value from several measured or binomial variables	Multiple linear regression or nonlinear regression (Example-21)	—	Multiple logistic regression (Example-22)

(ANOVA: analysis of variance)

were given the drug for 1 week, and the difference in blood pressure was measured after the treatment compared to the baseline value.

- *Null hypothesis (H0):* The mean reduction in blood pressure is equal to 10 mm Hg.
- *Alternative hypothesis (H1):* The mean reduction in blood pressure is not equal to 10 mm Hg.

EXAMPLE-2: WILCOXON RANK-SUM TEST

A clinical study aimed to detect the analgesic effect of—dexmedetomidine with ketamine, which was claimed to reduce pain score measured by VAS by 3 units *(qualitative—ordinal variable)*. The study involved 50 patients who were given the medications. After a specified period, the patients rated their pain relief on a scale from 1 to 10, with 10 denoting complete relief.

- *Null hypothesis (H0):* The median reduction in pain relief scores (VAS) is equal to 3 units.
- *Alternative hypothesis (H1):* The median reduction in pain relief scores (VAS) is not equal to 3 units.

EXAMPLE-3: PEARSON'S CHI-SQUARE TEST

A newer vaccine was rolled out for Monkeypox disease and its efficacy was claimed to be 90% *(proportion or nominal data)*. This vaccine was administered to 1,000 healthcare workers at a health centre and its efficacy (absence or presence of disease) was computed.

- *Null hypothesis (H0):* The proportion of health workers protected from Monkeypox is equal to 90%.
- *Alternative hypothesis (H1):* The proportion of health workers protected from Monkeypox is not equal to 90%.

EXAMPLE-4: UNPAIRED T-TEST

A study was performed to compare the blood pressure levels lowered by a newly introduced antihypertensive drug (ARNI). The drug was administered to one arm of patients, while the other arm received conventional treatment (beta-blocker) and the difference in mm Hg *(quantitative—continuous variable)* was computed and compared.

- *Null hypothesis (H0):* There is no difference in reduction of blood pressure between both drugs.
- *Alternative hypothesis (H1):* There is significant difference in reduction of blood pressure between both drugs.

EXAMPLE-5: MANN-WHITNEY U TEST

A study compared the analgesic effect of two drug combinations—dexmedetomidine with ketamine in one group and propofol with ketamine in another group and the outcome was measurement of pain score using VAS *(qualitative—ordinal variable).*

- *Null hypothesis (H0):* The median reduction in pain relief scores (VAS) is equal in both groups.
- *Alternative hypothesis (H1):* The median reduction in pain relief scores (VAS) is not equal in both groups.

EXAMPLE-6: FISHER'S EXACT CHI-SQUARE TEST

A study was conducted to compare the effect of newer antibiotic (Group A) in reducing the postoperative infections following total knee replacement (TKR) surgery when compared to the conventional antibiotic treatment (Group B). The proportion of patients without infection *(proportion or nominal data)* was compared between the groups. Fisher's exact was applied in place of Pearson's Chi-square when the expected cell count was <5 in >20% of cells in a contingency table.

- *Null hypothesis (H0):* The proportion of patients getting infected is equal in both the groups.
- *Alternative hypothesis (H1):* The proportion of patients getting infected is significantly different in both the groups.

EXAMPLE-7: PAIRED T-TEST

In a study among pregnant mothers, Hb% *(paired continuous variable)* was calculated before and after administration of iron and folic acid tablets and the values were compared.

- *Null hypothesis (H0):* The Hb% levels are equal before and after intervention.
- *Alternative hypothesis (H1):* The Hb% levels are significantly different before and after intervention.

EXAMPLE-8: WILCOXON TEST

A study was conducted to determine the analgesic effect of an epidural anaesthetic administered at the time of delivery. It was measured by pain score (using VAS) at 0 hour and 4 hours post-delivery *(paired ordinal data).*

- *Null hypothesis (H0):* The median pain score (VAS) is equal at both time intervals.
- *Alternative hypothesis (H1):* The median pain score (VAS) is not equal at both time intervals.

EXAMPLE-9: MCNEMAR'S TEST

A study was conducted to identify pancreatic cancer using computed tomography (CT) and magnetic resonance imaging (MRI) scan in a set of patients and the outcome was presence or absence of tumour *(paired nominal data).*

- *Null hypothesis (H0):* There is no difference in diagnostic accuracy between both the investigations.
- *Alternative hypothesis (H1):* There is a difference in diagnostic accuracy between both the investigations.

EXAMPLE-10: ONE-WAY ANALYSIS OF VARIANCE

In a trial, the anti-inflammatory effects of three drugs A, B, and C were compared by measuring the C-reactive protein (CRP) levels *(≥3 unpaired continuous variable).*

- *Null hypothesis (H0):* The CRP levels are equal in all the intervention groups.
- *Alternative hypothesis (H1):* The CRP levels are significantly different between the intervention groups.

EXAMPLE-11: KRUSKAL–WALLIS ANALYSIS OF VARIANCE TEST

A study was conducted to determine the analgesic effect of three drugs A, B, and C administered preoperatively to tonsillectomy patients. The outcome was measured by pain score (using VAS scale) after surgery in all the three groups *(≥3 unpaired ordinal data).*

- *Null hypothesis (H0):* The median pain scores (VAS) are equal in all the intervention groups
- *Alternative hypothesis (H1):* The median pain scores (VAS) are significantly different between the intervention groups.

EXAMPLE-12: PEARSON'S CHI-SQUARE TEST

A study recruited three groups. Group A was given Paleo diet, group B was given Mediterranean diet, and group C was asked to follow intermittent fasting for a period of 6 weeks. The outcome was presence or absence of weight loss in all the groups *(≥3 unpaired nominal data).*

- *Null hypothesis (H0):* The proportion of persons losing weight is similar in all the three groups.
- *Alternative hypothesis (H1):* The proportions of persons losing weight are significantly different in all the three groups.

EXAMPLE-13: REPEATED MEASURES ANALYSIS OF VARIANCE

A clinical trial aimed to determine if a new antihypertensive medication was effective in reducing the blood pressure over time. The study involved 100 patients who were randomly assigned to two groups: Group A received the new medication, and Group B received a placebo. Blood pressure levels were measured in mm Hg at four different time points: before the treatment, 1 week, 2 weeks, and 4 weeks after the treatment *(≥ 3 paired continuous variable).*

- *Null hypothesis (H0):* There is no significant difference in the mean blood pressure levels between the new medication and the placebo at any of the time points.
- *Alternative hypothesis (H1):* There is a significant difference in the mean blood pressure levels between the new medication and the placebo at one or more of the time points.

EXAMPLE-14: FRIEDMAN TEST

A clinical trial tested the effectiveness of three different analgesic techniques (A, B, and C) used in postoperative care. The study enroled 30 patients randomly assigned to three groups. Group A received Technique A, Group B received Technique B, and Group C received Technique C. Pain levels were measured on a VAS of 1–10 at three different time points: immediately after surgery, 24 hours post-surgery, and 48 hours post-surgery *(≥3 paired ordinal data).*

- *Null hypothesis (H0):* There is no significant difference in the median pain levels among the three pain management techniques at any of the time points.
- *Alternative hypothesis (Ha):* There is a significant difference in the median pain levels among the three pain management techniques at one or more of the time points.

EXAMPLE-15: COCHRANE-Q

This is an extension of McNemar's test that can be applied when three or more related (paired) proportions are compared. In a tertiary centre, the subjects who had come for cardiac screening were advised to undergo—electrocardiography, 2D-echocardiography, treadmill test, and CT coronary angiography to rule out any abnormalities. The outcome was the presence or absence of any abnormalities *(≥3 paired nominal data).*

- *Null hypothesis (H0):* There is no difference in diagnostic accuracy between the screening methods.
- *Alternative hypothesis (H1):* There is a difference in diagnostic accuracy between at least one or more screening methods.

EXAMPLE-16: PEARSON'S CORRELATION COEFFICIENT

In a study, the researchers aimed to determine the correlation between blood pressure (in mm Hg) and heart rate (beats per minute) in patients with hypertension *(comparing two normally distributed continuous data).*

- *Null hypothesis (H0):* If the calculated "r" value is close to "0", there is no significant correlation between blood pressure and heart rate.
- *Alternative hypothesis (H1):* If the calculated "r" value is close to "1" or "–1", it indicates a strong positive or negative correlation respectively.

EXAMPLE 17: SPEARMAN'S CORRELATION COEFFICIENT

When the data does not follow a normal distribution or when the relationship between variables is not linear, the Spearman's correlation coefficient ρ (rho) is used. In one study, the correlation between preoperative anxiety scoring (VAS score) with postoperative uterine cramping pain (VAS score) was measured 8 hours post-surgery.

- *Null hypothesis (H0):* If the calculated "ρ" value is close to "0", there is no significant correlation between anxiety and pain.
- *Alternative hypothesis (H1):* If the calculated "ρ" value is close to "1" or "–1", it indicates a strong positive or negative correlation respectively.

EXAMPLE-18: SIMPLE LINEAR REGRESSION

This will be an extension of Pearson's correlation coefficient (Example-16) where one is going to find the strength and direction of linear relationship between two quantitative variables (Example: Body mass index (BMI)—an independent variable and blood pressure—a dependent variable). In regression, for any given value of independent variable (x), one can predict the value of the dependent variable (y) using the linear regression model that derives a linear equation ($y = mx + a$). In this formula, "m" is the slope that will be represented by "β" in the model and "a" is the constant. Furthermore, the model predicts the measure of variance in the dependent variable that is denoted by coefficient of determination (R^2). The result will be measured and displayed as "β" or the slope with 95% CI and it is comprehended as follows. If the "β" value is 2.5 with 95% CI 1.7–3.9, then the inference will be that for every unit (kg/m^2) rise of BMI, the blood pressure will rise by 2.5 mm Hg on an average and if this is repeated in 100 samples, the value will be lying between 1.7 and 3.9 in 95 samples (95%).

Nonlinear regression is used in cases wherein a quantity decreases at a rate proportional to the existing value. For example, the rate at which a drug is excreted (t1/2) is proportional to the amount of drug present, an equation is derived and one can predict the amount of drug that will be present at any given point of time.

EXAMPLE 19: NONPARAMETRIC REGRESSION

This method is used if a researcher wants to predict the outcome (dependent variable) using input (independent variable or risk factor), knowing that the relationship between two quantitative variables is nonlinear. For example, blood pressure increases with age to a certain extent and it falls down, thus giving an inverted "U"-shaped relationship, and for prediction, one has to construct a fitting curve or apply locally weighted scatterplot smoothing (LOWESS) technique. The smoothing degree is assessed and a smooth curve will be created with the data points. Thereby, this model will be robust even when the outliers are present.

EXAMPLE 20: SIMPLE LOGISTIC REGRESSION

When the relationship between septic shock (present or absent), an independent variable, and the survival (yes or no), the dependent variable is established using Pearson's Chi-square test or Fisher's exact Chi-square test, the next step would be to predict the risk of survival in patients with septic shock. In such a case, the simple logistic regression model is used. The results will be measured in "OR" or "RR" along with 95% CI.

EXAMPLE 21: MULTIPLE LINEAR REGRESSION

This is applicable when the goal is to model the relationship of multiple predictor variables and the response variable and both are measured in interval or ratio scale (quantitative variables). In continuation with Example 18, there would be multiple predictors of blood pressure other than BMI such as total calorie intake (kcal per day), duration of physical activity (hours) or metabolic equivalents (METS) spent, etc. and all of these would be affecting the blood pressure. Hence, this regression adjusts the effects of all variables, meaning, it gives the more accurate relationship of only BMI with blood pressure, only total calorie intake and blood pressure, etc., adjusting the other variables. Thus, we get the adjusted "β" value and 95% CI for each independent variable (predictor).

EXAMPLE 22: MULTIPLE LOGISTIC REGRESSION

This is applicable when the goal is to model the relationship of multiple predictor variables and the response variable and both are measured in proportions. If cervical cancer (present or absent) is taken as the outcome and the factors such as HPV vaccination (taken or not), recurrent pelvic inflammatory disease (yes or no), early menarche (yes or no), etc. that are found associated by Pearson's Chi-square test, multiple logistic regression analysis has to be performed to evaluate if these variables predict the incidence of cervical cancer individually by adjusting the effects of other variables. We thus get adjusted OR or RR with 95% CI.

SPECIAL POINTS TO UNDERSTAND

- *Mantel–Haenszel test:* Mantel–Haenszel test is used to analyse the relationship between two categorical variables while controlling for a third variable (confounding factor). For example, if the association between gestational diabetes mellitus (GDM) (group—diabetic/nondiabetic) and the mode of delivery (outcome group—lower segment caesarean section(LSCS)/normal vaginal delivery) is calculated while controlling for BMI (a potential confounder), we should use the Mantel–Haenszel test to determine if the association between GDM and LSCS remains significant after accounting for BMI as a confounding variable.

- *F-value in analysis of variance (ANOVA):* It compares the variance between the groups to that within the groups. Higher F-value indicates that the groups differ from each other significantly in terms of the mean values, while a low F-value suggests the differences are likely due to chance and this will be accompanied by a *p*-value by which one can get the inference.
- *R^2 in regression analysis:* It is a statistical measure representing the proportion of variance in the dependent variable (y) that can be explained by that in the independent variable (x) in a regression model. Higher R-squared indicates that a model is better fit, meaning the model can explain well about the larger portion of variation of dependent variable while a lower R-squared explains poor fit and that the model is able to predict only smaller portion of variation of the dependent variable.

SECTION 7 SURVIVAL ANALYSIS

Table 7 provides a concise guide to selecting appropriate statistical methods for survival data, where the outcome is time until an event (e.g., death, relapse, and recovery).

TIME-TO-EVENT DATA

Time-to-event data or survival data, record the time taken for a specific event to take place. In medical terms, it refers to time taken for a complication, disease progression, or death to occur in a given time period. It helps us in evaluating the effectiveness of treatments and identifying the prognostic factors.

Most of the times, the individuals either drop out of a study or the study ends before the event occurs and this is called "censoring" and is a key characteristic of time-to-event data.

KAPLAN–MEIER SURVIVAL CURVE

Let us begin with an example. A clinical trial recruited patients with carcinoma prostate into two groups, with one receiving standard treatment and the other receiving the new treatment. The primary outcome was survival after 100 months of treatment. Here, the time-to-event will be—time from the diagnosis to death or end of the 100 months study period. Patients who are still alive at the end of the study period will be considered to be "censored". Observe the **Figure 19**. The "black line" denotes the standard treatment while the "gray line" denotes the new treatment group. The steep curve (for black line) indicates increased

TABLE 7: Common statistical tests and models used in survival analysis.

Groups	*Survival time or survival analysis (measurements)*
One group	Kaplan–Meier survival curve
Comparison of two unpaired groups	Log–Rank test
Comparison of two paired groups	Conditional proportional hazard regression
Comparison of three or more unmatched groups	Cox proportional hazard regression
Comparison of three or more matched groups	Conditional proportional hazard regression
Prediction of value from another measured variable	Cox proportional hazard regression
Prediction of value from several measured or binomial variables	Cox proportional hazard regression

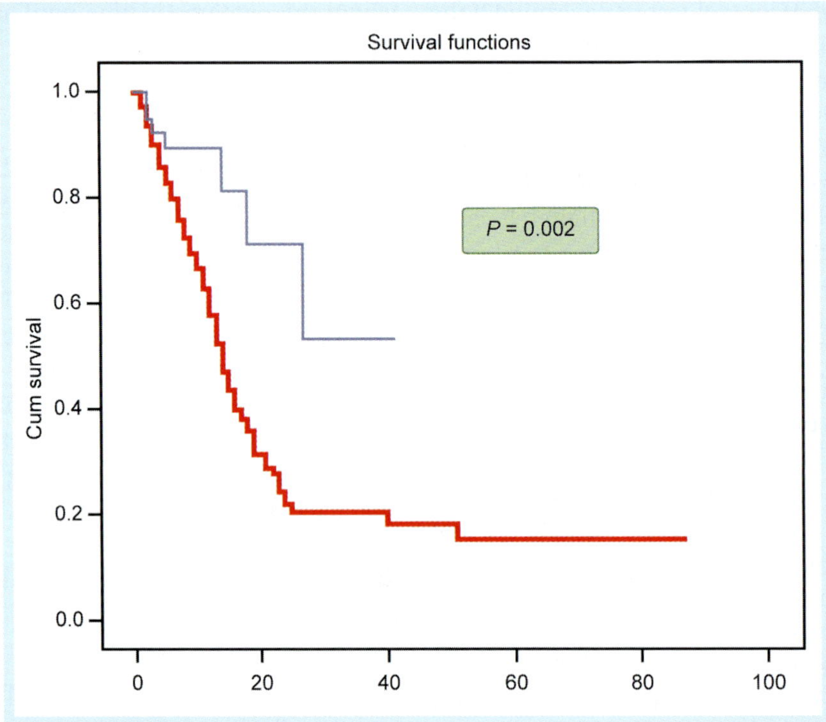

Fig. 19: Kaplan-Meier survival curve

mortality in that group compared to that in the new treatment group. If the curve crosses at any point in-between the study period, it means the survival experiences of the groups differ at different time points. The horizontal steps indicate the changes in probability of survival that generally occur at the time of observed events or censoring.

LOG-RANK TEST

This compares the survival distributions of two or more groups; for instance, the survival times of patients with carcinoma colon (after surgery) in two treatment groups—Group A (only chemotherapy) and Group B (chemoradiation). We collect data on the time of death or last follow-up for each patient in both groups. We then use the Log-Rank test to determine if there is a significant difference in survival times between Group A and Group B. The test calculates a *p*-value, which tells us if the difference in survival times is statistically significant or if it could have occurred by chance. Thereby, the effectiveness of the treatments in prolonging survival for patients in each group can be assessed.

COX PROPORTIONAL HAZARDS REGRESSION

In continuation with the example for Log-Rank test, apart from treatment, there might be other factors (covariates) such as age, gender, stage of cancer, comorbidities, etc. that might influence the survival of carcinoma colon patients. This model specifies the intervention group as the primary predictor and covariates as additional predictors.

This regression gives us the "HRs", i.e., hazard associated with the intervention group and the covariates compared to the control group. A HR >1 indicates higher risk of mortality for the intervention group or higher values of covariates and vice-versa. Cox proportional hazards regression assumes that the HR between two individuals remains constant over time. This means that the RR of an event occurring at a specific time does not change based on the values of covariates.

CONDITIONAL PROPORTIONAL HAZARDS REGRESSION

Conditional proportional hazards regression extends the Cox proportional hazards model to allow for *time-varying covariates*. This means that the HR can change over time based on the values of these covariates. If in the above study, evaluating the effect of a new treatment for colon cancer and the treatment's effectiveness remains constant over time, a Cox proportional hazards regression model would be appropriate. However, if the effectiveness of treatment changes based on a patient's weight or immune status, which might fluctuate over time, a conditional proportional hazards regression model would be necessary to account for the time-varying covariate (weight or immunity status).

CONCLUSION

- Understanding how to categorise data as qualitative or quantitative is foundational for choosing appropriate statistical methods in biostatistics.
- Tools like frequency tables, bar charts, and proportions help to summarise and visualise discrete variables, thereby aiding in the clear interpretation of health trends.
- Measures such as mean, median, variance, and histograms provide insights into numerical data distributions essential for analysing biological measurements.
- Grasping probability models enables the prediction of outcomes in uncertain biological events, forming the basis for inferential statistics.
- Effective screening tests balance sensitivity and specificity to detect diseases early, improving the outcomes of diagnostic tests and the overall upliftment of public health.
- Assessing inter-rater reliability through kappa statistics ensures consistency in diagnostic or observational data between the physicians.
- ROC curves evaluate diagnostic test performance and help in the selection of optimal thresholds for accuracy. One can thereby determine the cut-off values for presence or absence of disease apart from grading the disease severity.
- CIs and point estimates quantify population parameters from samples, incorporating core concepts like sampling error.
- Hypothesis tests, p-values, and t-tests determine if observed differences in data are statistically meaningful and thus guide evidence-based decisions.
- Methods like Kaplan-Meier curves and Cox models analyse time-to-event data, crucial for studying patient outcomes in clinical trials.

BIBLIOGRAPHY

1. Banerjee B. Mahajan's methods in biostatistics for medical students and research workers. 9th ed. New Delhi: Jaypee Brothers Medical Publishers; 2018.
2. Bhalwar, R. Textbook of Public Health and Community Medicine, Published in Collaboration with WHO. Department of Community Medicine, AFMC, Pune; 2009.
3. Le CT, Eberly LE. Introductory Biostatistics. 2nd ed. Hoboken (NJ): John Wiley & Sons;2016.
4. Nafis F. Biostatistics Manual for Health Research: A Practical Guide to Data Analysis. Oxford, UK: Academic Press; 2023.
5. Park K. Park's Textbook of Preventive and Social Medicine. 27th ed. Jabalpur: Banarsidas Bhanot Publishers; 2023.
6. Petrie A, Sabin C. Medical statistics at a glance. 4th ed. Hoboken, NJ: Wiley-Blackwell; 2020.

9

CHAPTER

Data Collection and Representation of Data in the Graphical Format

Nishant Sahay, Prashant Joshi

INTRODUCTION

Genius is 1% inspiration and 99% perspiration, so is the postgraduate thesis or dissertation. The 1% here refers to designing the study protocol, aims and objectives, flow charts, trial registration, the patient information sheets and the consent forms, which are essential to document the intent and purpose of the study. Very soon, artificial intelligence models will likely prepare these in no time. Then starts the 99%: executing what we set out to do. This includes data collection, representation, analysis and interpretation. Each step is as critical as the rest. Poor data collection and handling can directly impact the study results and lead to distrust in the claims being made. Improper representation of collected data leads to inefficient communication. In this chapter, we touch upon various aspects pertaining to data collection and representation.

DATA MANAGEMENT

Data is the new oil. One must have heard this statement used exceedingly in the context of geopolitics, especially because of the explosion of good quality, reliable, and near real-time data which gets collected across the globe through satellites, cameras, and personal digital devices.[1] Countries and companies which own this data can glean incredible insight into myriad domains and use it for their benefit. It is so much more useful because there is a lot of automation in the data collection and most of it is done by machines which have been created for this exclusive purpose. The data that we collect in medical sciences, however, for the context of this textbook, during our postgraduate thesis, does not entirely fall into the automated data collection category.[2] Sure, there are digital, connected, and smart machines which measure parameters of our interest hands-off, but there is still a significant component of human setup and oversight required in these to make the data collection reliable. We also want to share this data with our peers, who may want to replicate our study and see if our findings hold true in a different context (such as different geography, climate, gender, age group, etc.), so we need to report as much details of our data collection procedure as is relevant and possible so as to facilitate these replication studies. This basic intent forms the crux of the different processes one needs to follow while collecting, storing, analysing, and reporting the data, so that it serves the purpose of our scientific endeavour. Can the process be perfect though? It seldom is, despite all the best laid plans of man...as the saying goes. The best we can do is to plan for the known variables which affect our parameter of interest and try to be accurate each time we collect the data for that parameter. Unknown influences can always affect the data; therefore, it is important to describe in detail the methodology with which the data was collected.[3] After the entire data collection, we can look at the distribution and check if any outliers are there, which may skew our measures of central tendencies.[4] *Description* and *disclosure* are the way to go and these should be well written in the "Material and Methods" section of the thesis document. Details of the *material* used are equally important, it could be the make of the machine, the technology used, the specific way a buffer was prepared, or something as simple as whether the blood pressure was measured in a sitting or a sleeping posture. Each of these parameters can affect the measured data, therefore they form an important part of the setting to be described.

With this context, let us look at some of the best practices to collect and manage our data.

DATA COLLECTION

Types of Data

Qualitative versus Quantitative Data

- *Qualitative data:* Nominal and descriptive non-numerical data cannot be measured. This kind of data is usually encountered in studies which are interview-based or involve a component of surveys.[5] To make this kind of data collection robust, we must use validated questionnaires and design the collection such that some internal measures of consistency are built in. These forms of data are also generally difficult to summarise and do not apply to the larger general population very well.
- Quantitative data, on the other hand, can be easily summarised and be generalised well, given the study has been designed with an adequate power and confidence level. The mathematical language we use in these studies is well suited to convey the extent of limitations of our findings.

Primary versus Secondary Data

- *Primary data collection* is the data which is being collected directly from the subject/participant of interest.[6] Most of our medical postgraduate theses are designed to collect primary data, because this makes the student encounter the process of data collection, its challenges and vicissitudes, such that a visceral understanding of this process develops. This helps us critically analyse the published scientific data and evaluate in our own context. Some of the important things to keep in mind for primary data collection are:
  - Check the accuracy level and validity of the instrument used for collection [thermometer, blood pressure monitor, automated machines, sensors, etc.]. If a regular calibration and audit of the equipment is being done at the centre, it is useful to state it in the methodology as a quality assurance parameter.[7]
  - Describe and note and be aware of enough parameters which can account for systemic differences in the parameter of interest.
  - *Standardise and report the methodology in detail:* Staining methods, buffer preparation, etc. Use internationally accepted terminologies and classification criteria wherever applicable.
  - *Real-time data collection versus collection from archival material/case sheets:* This depends on the study design and each has its own challenges. Typically, the study designs of each medical college department are limited in variation and therefore it helps to gain some understanding of how best to execute a particular study design. A common study design in *anaesthesia,* for example, relates to the intraoperative haemodynamic parameters with a new drug or combination compared with the current accepted standard. The real-time data in this design needs to be collected on the operation theatre table as per previously defined time points. If we can automate the data collection process through the monitors, the reliability of data increases as it reduces logistical as well as transcription errors. Automated data collection thus is also a way of quality assurance.[2] A common study design in pathology is based on assessment of

an immunomarker expression or any histological scoring system in a tumour of particular type. This is generally based on archival tissue which is retrieved for the study purpose. In this context, the best practice to ensure data robustness varies, for e.g., immunomarker expression in archival tissues, especially those not stored properly, can be markedly less, compared to recent cases. The quality of chemicals used in processing also varies over time, so these factors need to be considered such that all the cases included are at an equal footing, with respect to the parameter of interest.

- *Prevent manual/transcription errors:* Especially important when a range of people are involved in collecting the primary data. Consider use of digital data collection tools to minimise these errors.[8]
- Use reproducible methods, or methods and scoring systems which have good reported intra- and interobserver variability.
- *Subjective parameters:* Define methodology as much as possible to allow reproducibility, report inter- and intraobserver variation wherever possible.
- *Collect, store, and share complete and valid metadata:* Especially in relation to digital images. They are usually collected as default by most devices. It is important to store a set of original images which are not being modified in any way for either thesis document or journal article publication.[9]
- Why should I believe your data is true and not made up? A lot of this runs on trust since it is impractical to independently verify every single data point being collected. However, in cases where disputes are raised or complaints received, institutional mechanisms require that primary evidence be produced to back the claims made in any thesis or manuscript under consideration. Many universities have set up administrative structures to investigate possible research fraud and poor data collection, storage, and management that can reflect poorly on the research team and can have devastating career implications.[10] Software which facilitates data entry and tracks modifications can be useful tools of quality assurance. One such tool is REDCap (https://projectredcap.org/).[11] In this context, it is important to maintain a chain of verification for the data being noted. Reversibly coded data should be verifiable, if the need arises (e.g., machine readings archival data backup, patient case records, video recordings, slides and blocks, and original digital images without any modifications).

- *Secondary data:* This is the data which already exists in some form (journal articles, abstracts, tumour registries, etc.) and is being compiled and analysed with a particular objective in mind. Typically, *systematic reviews, narrative reviews,* and *meta-analyses,* increasingly used in medical science over the past few decades, are all analyses of secondary data.[6] As a researcher interested in performing such an analysis, it is important to learn how to frame a specific research objective and then gather data from all possible sources to be compiled and analysed. It is important to define the search strategy such that it covers the most resources and apply it uniformly across all databases to begin with. There are many resources on the internet which summarise these points well (e.g., Cochrane.org) and need to be followed to ensure a good quality secondary analysis.
- *Missing data:* These are the data points which were planned to be collected, however, could not be during the stipulated course of the research project. If it is an important variable,

the cases with missing data and the way they were dealt with should be reported, including the reasons for missing data. In some research areas, artificial values are imputed in these missing data points, but for biomedical studies it is best not to do so.[12] The statistician should also be made aware of this.

Data Validation

- Predefined quality criteria should be set for including the data for further analysis.
- Data points which do not meet the quality criteria (measurement errors, inaccuracies, and not fitting inclusion criteria on review) should be removed. This does not always mean removing the outliers.
- It forms part of cleaning the data before proceeding for analysis.[13] In some kinds of data, for example, genomic data derived from next generation sequencers, some of these steps are well defined and standardised. One way to assess the quality of reads being generated is through a "Phred score" which determines the probability of error at a single nucleotide level. It is routine in these analyses to remove all the reads with a Phred score below a certain threshold.[14]
- Best practices to keep data safe include:
    - Digital entry with backups (local drives or cloud based). It is important to look for services adhering to health insurance portability and accountability act (HIPAA) compliance standards to maintain the privacy, security, and integrity of patients' protected health information.[15]
    - Always retain the original unedited high resolution digital images with their meta data.
    - Hard copy backup, best pasted in the thesis hard copies.
    - Password protect data master chart to prevent ungranted access and theft.

REPRESENTATION OF DATA IN THE GRAPHICAL FORMAT

Data is any information in the raw or organised form. One can use alphabets, numbers, or even symbols that refer to or represent objects, preferences, ideas, traits, categories, etc., and it is important to interpret these symbols, numbers, and alphabets into something meaningful. Once data has been obtained, an easily comprehensible representation in the form of graphs, figures, or tables, facilitates quick interpretations and instant understanding.

We have seen that data can be of different types, qualitative or quantitative. Qualitative data is also called categorical, frequency counts, or descriptive data because they approximate, characterise, and measure attributes.[16] These data cannot be measured as numbers, e.g., yes/no, colours, gender, etc. Qualitative data can be nominal, meaning described as names where there is no implication of order or ratio. Qualitative data, however, may convey an order or hierarchy and they are then said to be ordinal. The graphical representation of such data will be different from the data which may conveniently be described as numbers, i.e., the quantitative data.

Quantitative data are data in the form of counts or numbers where each dataset has a unique numerical value associated with it.[5]

Interval data: Numerical data which may be placed in a meaningful order having meaningful intervals between items, are said to be present on an interval scale, e.g., temperature measured in Celsius.[17]

Ratio scale: Some quantitative data in addition to being placed in a meaningful order with meaningful intervals between items, also have an absolute zero, and thus for these data, meaningful ratios also do exist. These data are said to be on a ratio scale. Most biomedical variables form a ratio scale: weight in grams or pounds, time in seconds or days, blood pressure in millimetres of mercury, and pulse rate in beats per minute are all ratio scale data. The temperature scale in Celsius is not a ratio scale. Here, as 0°C does not imply a complete absence of heat, a temperature of 100°C cannot be considered to be double of 50°C.[18]

Discrete data: When the variables can take only certain values and none in between and are expressed as a whole number, and not as fractions, e.g., number of patients in a hospital, the data is discrete data. On the other hand, data which can be represented as fractions of decimal numbers are called continuous data. Again, most biomedical variables are continuous data, e.g., a patient's weight, height, age, and blood pressure.[19]

Pictures speak a thousand words, and the human brain is remarkably adept in processing pictures easily. Pictographic or a graphical depiction of data can process large datasets in a relatively small space and also help in making large data more coherent. This facilitates easy and quick comparisons as the readers get a bird's eye view.

There are certain basic norms which must be kept in mind before converting data into graphs or diagrams.

- For representation on a graph, there are two axes that intersect each other at the "origin", depicted using "0,0".
- "X" axis, also called the abscissa (base) is the horizontal line. "Y" axis, the vertical line is called the ordinate (height). The ordinate/height/y-axis of the graph should be 75% of the abscissa/base/x-axis according to a 75% rule, but it may be flexible between 60% and 80%.
- Values of the abscissa (x-axis) toward the left of the origin (0) is negative (-) and similarly values of the ordinate (y-axis) below the origin is negative (-). The graph can thus be divided into four quadrants, and the quadrant having both positive values (++) is usually given the maximum space on a graph paper **(Fig. 1** and **Box 1)**.[20]

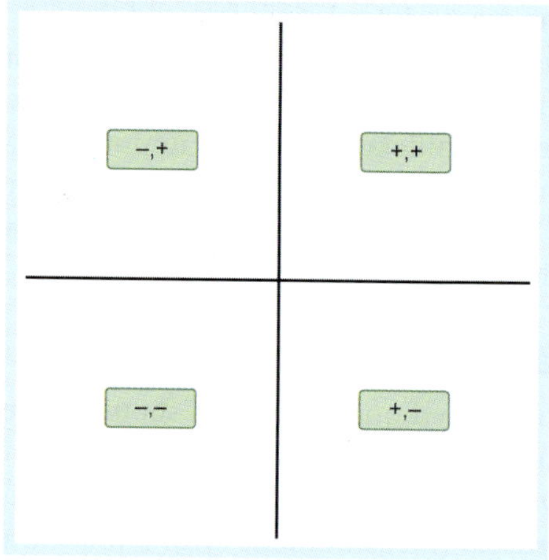

Fig. 1: Quadrants of a graph.

BOX 1: A basic template guiding graphical representation of data.

- Qualitative data
  - Line
  - Bar
    - Simple
    - Clustered
    - Stacked
  - Pie
  - Pictogram
  - Spot map
- Quantitative data
  - Histogram
  - Frequency polygon
  - Cumulative frequency polygon
  - Scatter diagram
  - Box and Whisker plot
  - Correlation diagram

TABLE 1: Month-wise sale of cars.

January	*February*	*March*	*April*	*May*	*June*
12	23	44	55	98	112

Line Chart/Graph (Table 1 and Fig. 2)

Line graphs or charts are mainly used to highlight trends or the changes of selected variables over time. Line graphs may be used for both discrete

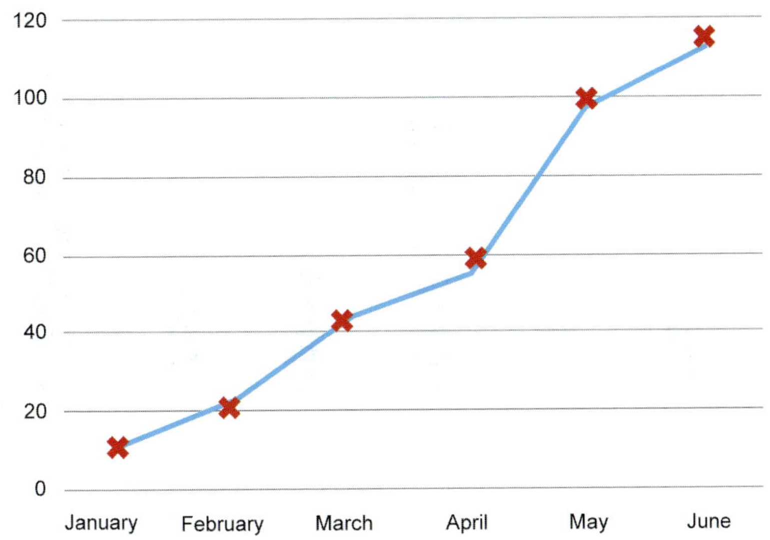

Fig. 2: Simple line graphical representation of sale of cars.

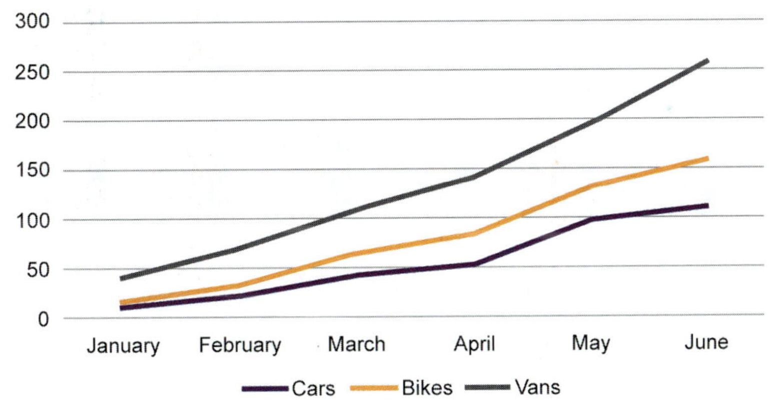

Fig. 3: Line graph showing sale of different vehicles.

and continuous data. The data values are crossed over at the appropriate coordinates along the x- and y-axis on the graph and connected by lines. This gives an instantaneous picture regarding the trends, e.g., month-wise sale of cars

The same line graph can also be used to compare different variables, e.g., sale of bikes, cars, and vans during the same time period. Each variable is marked in a different colour **(Fig. 3)**.

Bar Chart (Fig. 4)

Discrete data can be displayed in the form of a bar chart, especially if it is categorical data. The categorical data is often obtained as frequencies,

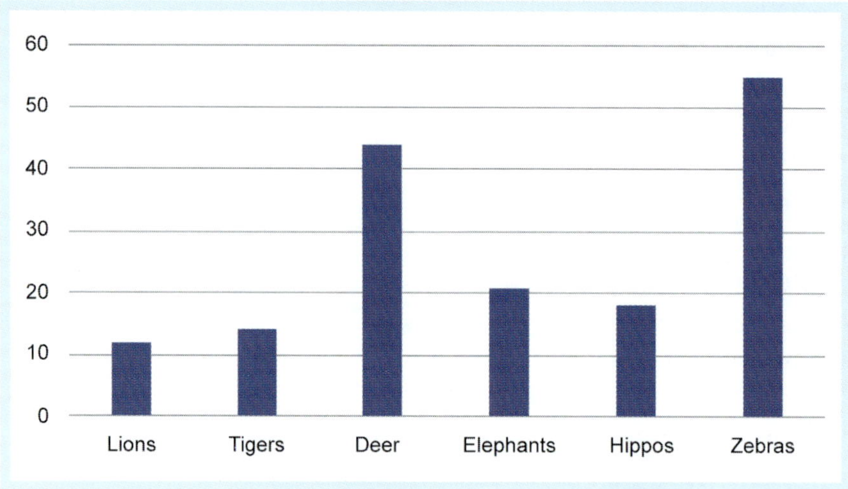

Fig. 4: Bar graph showing different animals in the zoo.

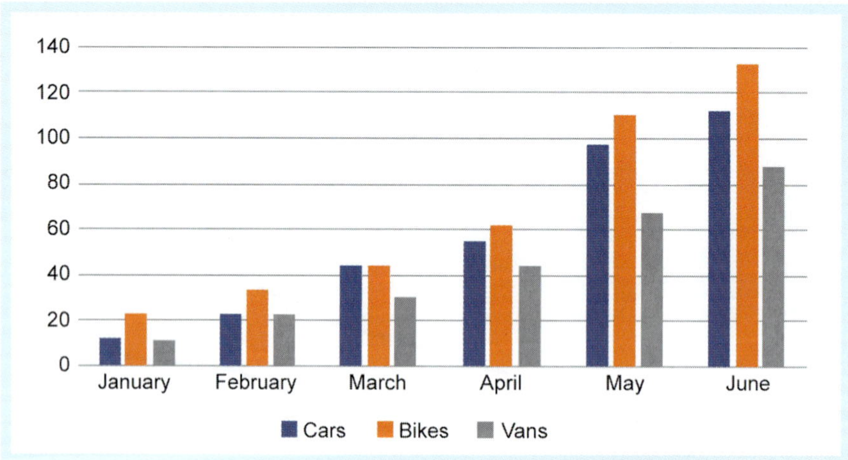

Fig. 5: Clustered bar chart showing vehicle sales.

e.g., animals in a zoo. This categorical data is then represented with bars with height proportional to the values that they represent. The bars can be plotted either vertically or horizontally. Chart with vertical bars is called a column chart. In any orientation, the bars should be evenly spaced and have the same width. The centre of the bar has discrete value or category. The frequencies are mostly placed along the y-axis.

Bar charts can be:

- Clustered or grouped bar charts
- Stacked or composite bar charts
- Variable width bar charts

Clustered bar charts have two or more colour-coded bars for each attribute, to represent a given data set, e.g., sales of many vehicles during a given time may be represented as in **Figure 5**.

Stacked bar charts, also called composite bar charts, stack the bars one on top of the other.[21] The height of each attribute reflects their individual contribution, and total length of each bar depicts the combined result. The same data set represented as a clustered bar chart earlier, has been represented as a stacked bar chart in **Figure 6**. Stacked bar charts help in a quick assessment of performance or trend of performance of the single variable **(Fig. 6)**.

Variable width charts are sometimes used to highlight differences in the categorical variable being studied, e.g., different countries with different populations contribute differently to global warming. In this figure, contribution to global pollution can thus be more realistically evaluated if assessed country-wise with total area of each bar representing the total contribution thereof **(Fig. 7)**.

Bar-line graphs are sometimes used to represent discrete data (e.g., number of students in a class, shirt size of students, etc.). A "bar-line chart" combines the advantages of bar charts and line graphs into a useful data visualisation tool. The bars typically represent discrete values or categories, displayed through rectangular

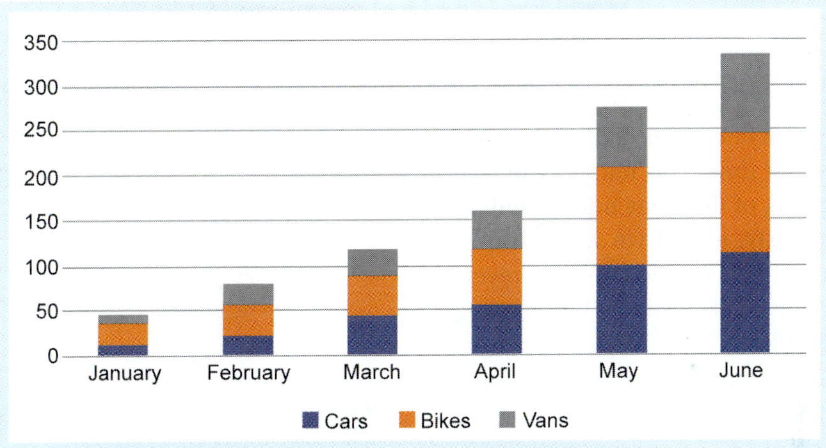

Fig. 6: Stacked bar charts showing vehicle sales in subsequent months.

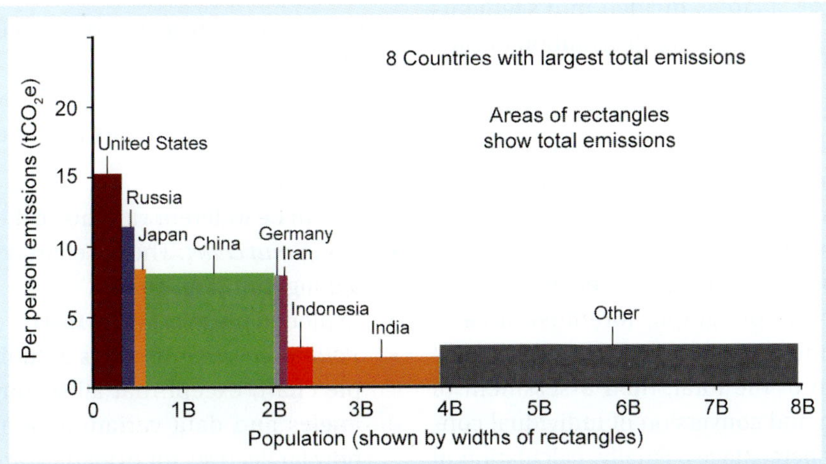

Fig. 7: Variable width bar charts showing carbon dioxide emissions per person.

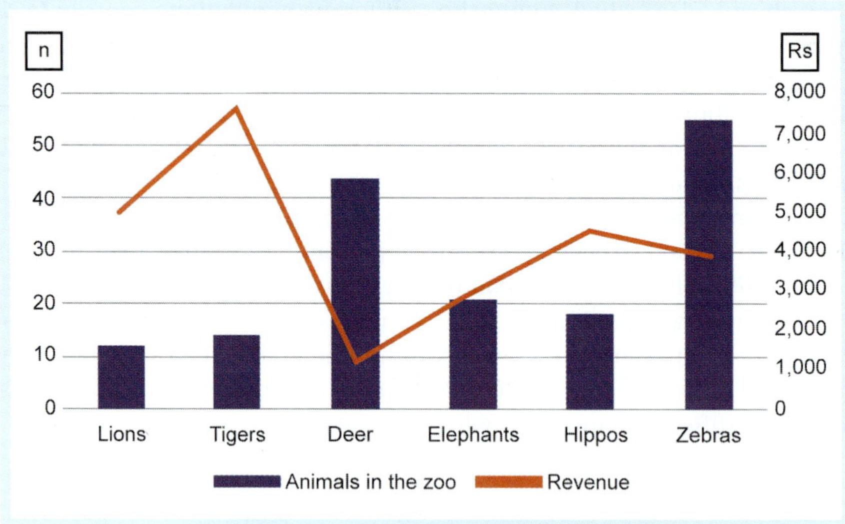

Fig. 8: Bar-line graph depicts the number (n) of animals in a zoo and the revenue these generate.

columns, while the line series shows continuous data or trends over time. This marriage of charts facilitates analysis of different but related data sets simultaneously, e.g., if we want to assess the number of animals in a zoo and the revenue generated per animal enclosure, a bar-line graph can be useful.[21] We can interpret that the revenue from deer is least despite them being greatest in numbers in a zoo **(Fig. 8)**.

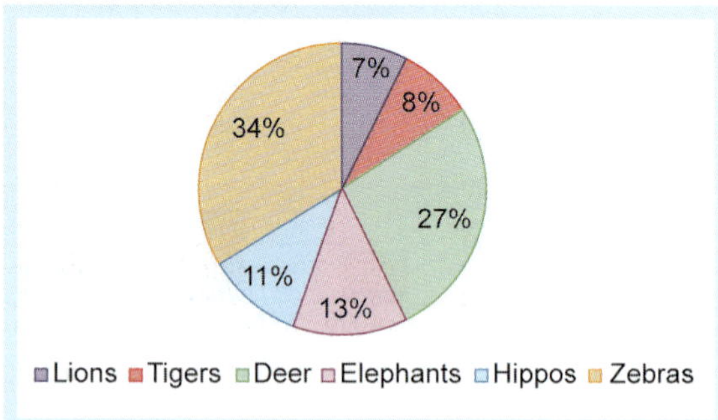

Fig. 9: Pie chart showing the animals in a zoo.

Pie Chart

A pie chart uses a circle, divided into segments or slices to depict the relative distribution of each category. The "pie" represents the whole, and the "slices" represent parts of the whole. The size of segments or the angle at the centre of each sector is proportional to the frequency. The number of sectors should, generally, not exceed 6–8 to make the presentation meaningful and allow comparison between the various sectors.

To create any pie graph, foremost, a categorisation of the data is needed. This is followed by calculation of the total, then assessment of categorisation and conversion of individual contribution into percentages. Finally, calculation of the angle to be subtended at the centre of the pie graph by each category is done to create the pie graph.[22]

An example of the pie chart representation for the number of animals in a zoo is shown in **Figure 9**.

There can be different variants of the pie chart.

- *Doughnut chart:* The pie chart is in the form of a doughnut **(Fig. 10A)**.
- Exploded pie chart **(Fig. 10B)**.
- *Polar area diagram:* This is similar to a usual pie chart, except that all sectors have equal angles and data variations are reflected by how far each sector extends from the centre of the circle **(Fig. 10C)**.[23]

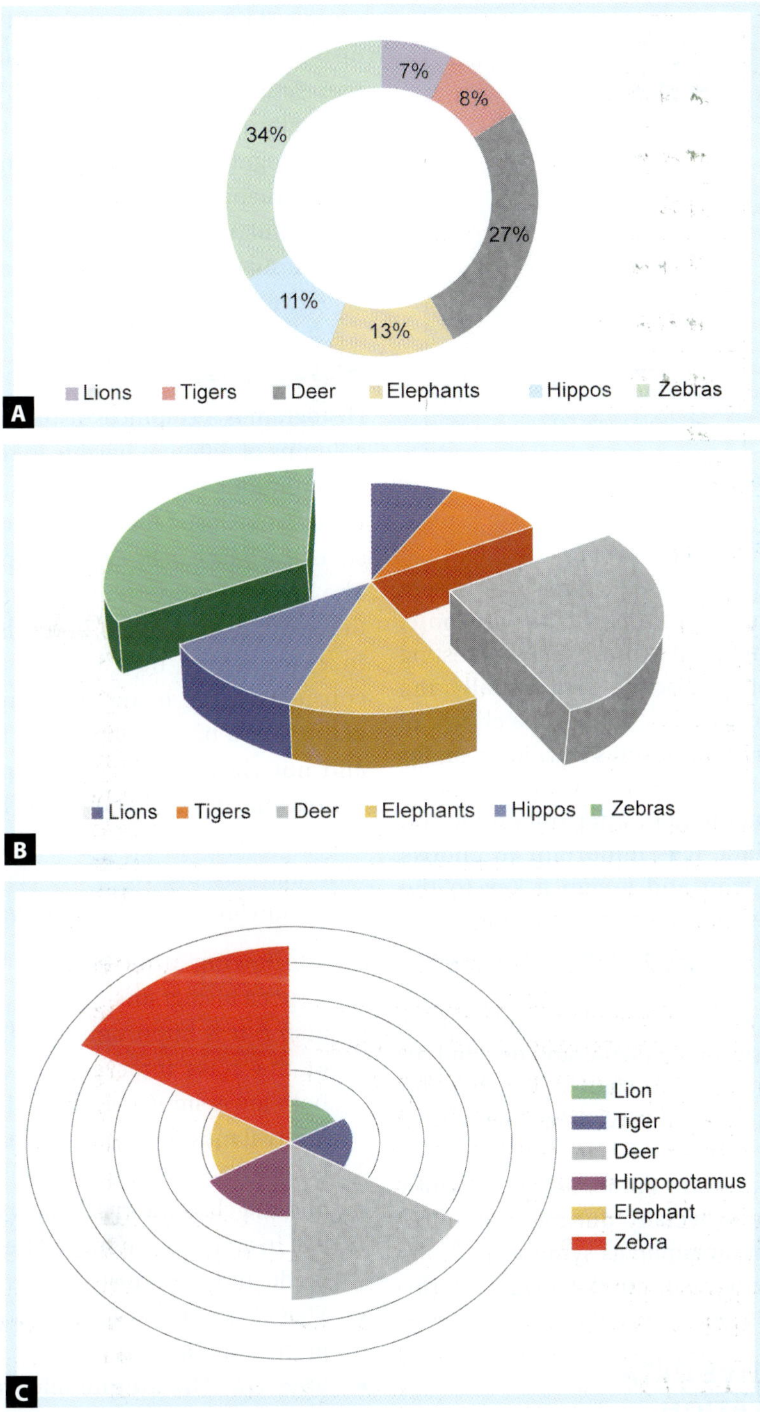

Figs. 10A to C: The variations of the pie charts.

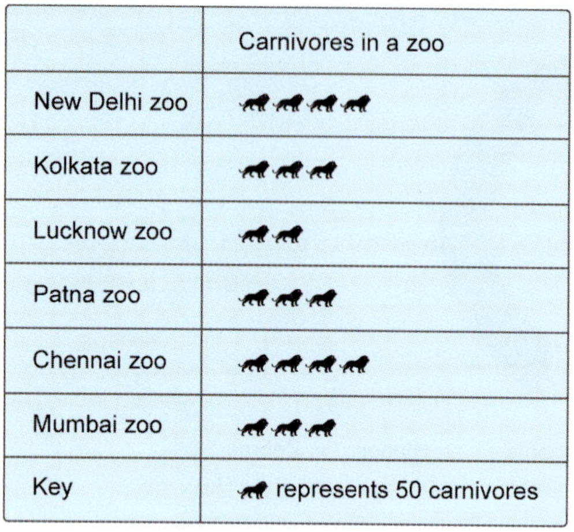

Fig. 11: Pictogram.

Pictograms (Fig. 11)

These are diagrams that use pictures to represent amounts or numbers of a particular attribute. Images or icons are used to present an interesting view of small sets of discrete data. Usually, the data attributes or category dictate the choice of icons, e.g., horse for herbivores and lion icon for carnivores.

To make a pictograph, after obtaining and reviewing the data, it is important to choose an appropriate icon and assign a key to the pictograph. Whilst drawing the pictograph, icons or any other symbol can also be represented as fractions if required. This will be needed when the frequency itself is not a whole number, or based upon the key of the pictograph decided. In the pictograph depicted in **Figure 11**, half a lion icon would mean 25 carnivores instead of the 50 as per key.

These are important epidemiological tools, used extensively especially during epidemics. Cases are plotted on a map as symbols or icons and then inferences about the origin of the epidemic and its mode of spread can be assessed.

QUANTITATIVE DATA REPRESENTATION

Quantitative data can be measured as a number. Continuous variables are those where data can be organised into class intervals and where frequency distribution tables can be prepared.[24] Graphical representation of such grouped, continuous data is usually done using any one of the following:

- Histogram or column diagrams
- Frequency polygons
- Cumulative frequency graphs
- Cumulative frequency percentage curves or ogives

Histograms

Histogram is a graphical display that uses vertical columns of different heights to represent data for a continuous variable, over a set of intervals. A histogram is used for continuous data where the statistical data can be arranged in class intervals.[25] The height is proportional to the frequency, and the width is dependent upon the class interval. In cases where bars of the same width are considered, the histogram may become a bar graph, but a bar graph is used for discrete data and not class intervals. For construction of a histogram, if data is given in inclusive series, data is converted into an exclusive series. It is customary to take two extra class intervals, one below and another above the given classes.

The following process may be followed to construct a histogram—

- *Step I:* It is important to calculate the limits of the class intervals. To compute limits, both lower limit and upper limit of each class interval must be found out, e.g., limits of class interval 5–9, will be 4.5 and 9.5, respectively, and the class interval is now depicted as 4.5–9.5. In an inclusive series, the limits should be made into an exclusive series.
- *Step II:* The lower limit and upper limits are plotted on the x-axis.
- *Step III:* The frequencies are plotted on the y-axis. Thereafter, each class interval is depicted using adjacent rectangular bars of equal width.

- *Step IV:* The selection of appropriate scales for both the x-axis and y-axis has to be kept in mind. Data as given in **Table 2** can be considered.

Following the steps, the histogram created will be as shown in **Figure 12**.

Bihistograms, made from two histograms in opposite directions, can be created by entering negative and positive data for the same interval values. Each half of the bihistogram represents a different category and can be back-to-back on opposite sides of either the y-axis or the x-axis. Bihistograms are a very useful way to compare skewness and outliers for two data categories.

TABLE 2: Data for graphical representation of grouped and continuous data.

Class interval	*Frequency*	*Class limit*
05–09	3	4.5–9.5
10–14	2	9.5–14.5
15–19	6	14.5–19.5
20–24	3	19.5–24.5
25–29	5	24.5–29.5
30–34	8	29.5–34.5

Frequency Polygons

These diagrams are sometimes used to represent data for a continuous variable, over a set of intervals. This is similar to the use of a histogram. The histogram and frequency polygons are both structured on similar graphs and on the same scales. Even the area covered by histogram bars and a frequency polygon created on the same set of data will be same. For construction of the frequency polygon, the midpoints of bars of the histogram may be joined. It is important to close the diagram by joining the ends of the lines to the x-axis by adding one class interval at the upper end and at the lower end of the distribution. On connecting the lines to the x-axis, the structure becomes a closed structure and is called the frequency polygon.[26]

For creation of the frequency polygon, let us assume the same data as given in **Table 3**.

The steps for creating a frequency polygon are as follows:

- *Step I:* Class intervals are assessed and the midpoints of class intervals are calculated and noted as (X).

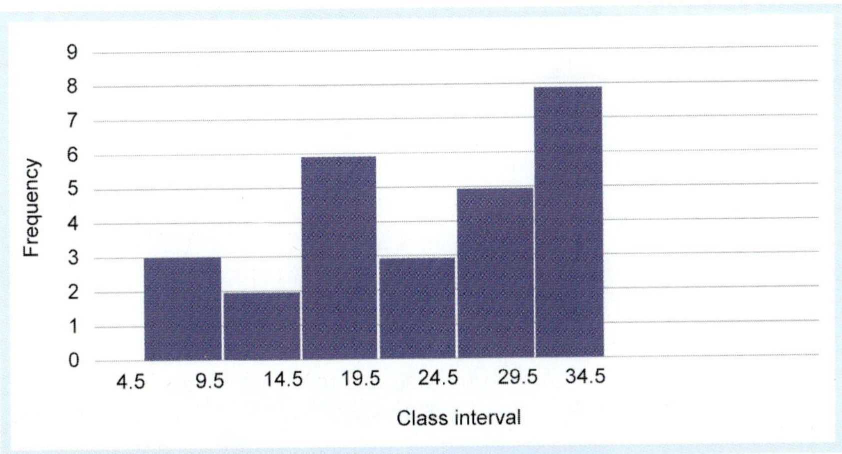

Fig. 12: Histogram showing class interval and frequency in each class.

- *Step II:* The midpoints of class intervals are represented on x-axis. The frequency of class intervals is indicated on y-axis.
- *Step III:* The corresponding frequencies are plotted against each midpoint in the graph and are connected using straight lines.
- *Step IV:* The midpoints of bars of the histogram may be joined. It is important to close the diagram by joining the ends of the lines to the x-axis by adding one class interval at upper end and at the lower end of the distribution **(Fig. 13)**.

Cumulative Frequency Polygon

To draw the cumulative frequency graph, an extra class interval is added at the lowest limit whose frequency is 0. Thereafter, the frequencies are added and thus the cumulative frequencies are found out **(Table 4)**.

The graph is now formed using the upper limit of class interval as the x-axis and the cumulative frequencies as the y-axis.

Cumulative Frequency Percentage Curve or Ogive Charts

The process of drawing the cumulative frequency percentage curve or ogive, is similar to cumulative frequency curve, except that, instead of the cumulative frequency, cumulative percentages are plotted along the y-axis. Upper limit of the class interval is the x-axis **(Table 5)**.

TABLE 3: Data for graphical representation.

Class interval	*Frequency*	*Cumulative frequency*
05–09	3	7
10–14	2	12
15–19	6	17
20–24	3	22
25–29	5	27
30–34	8	32

TABLE 4: Cumulative frequencies.

Class interval	*Frequency*	*Cumulative frequency*	*Upper limit of class interval*
00–04	0	0	4.5
05–09	3	3	9.5
10–14	2	5	14.5
15–19	6	11	19.5
20–24	3	14	24.5
25–29	5	19	29.5
30–34	8	27	34.5

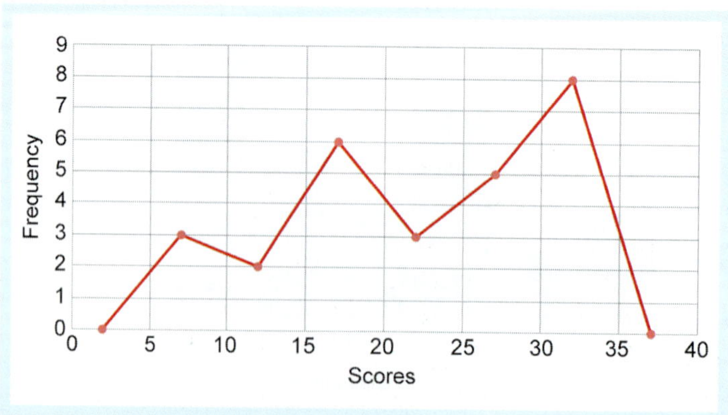

Fig. 13: Frequency polygon.

TABLE 5: Cumulative percentage.

Class interval	*Frequency*	*Cumulative frequency*	*% of cumulative frequency*	*Upper limit of class interval*
00–04	0	0	0	4.5
05–09	3	3	11	9.5
10–14	2	5	18	14.5
15–19	6	11	41	19.5
20–24	3	14	52	24.5
25–29	5	19	70	29.5
30–34	8	27	100	34.5

Utility of the *ogive* graphs lies in their ability to find the median of the given set of data. There are two types of *ogive* graphs which can be plotted using the same data asset. These are the "Less than" and "Greater than" cumulative frequency curves. When both are drawn on the same graph, the point at which both the curves intersect on the x-axis, is the median value. Ogives can also be used to know the percentiles of the data set values. The slope of the ogive curves also helps to quickly assess the rate of change of data points as one moves from one interval class to the next.

CONCLUSION

There can be more ways to depict data than discussed here, as newer methods are being tried for better data representation. To conclude, it must be reiterated that good data collection forms the core of a research study. Analyses and interpretations are only built around this core. Significant effort should be focused on this aspect so that the data that we collect is reliable and reproducible. Understanding the different ways of representing data helps us place our findings concisely and accurately. It provides a bird's-eye view of the data, facilitating more effective scientific communication and making a thesis more reader-friendly as well as easy to understand and comprehend.

REFERENCES

1. Quigley E, Holme I, Doyle DM, Ho AK, Ambrose E, Kirkwood K, et al. "Data is the new oil": citizen science and informed consent in an era of researchers handling of an economically valuable resource. Life Sciences, Society and Policy. 2021;17(1):9.
2. Snijkers G, Saraiva P, Van Wijk D, Martinez Solano JD, Rodrigues S. Automated business data collection: Experiences in Portugal and The Netherlands. Statistical Journal of the IAOS. 2025 Jun;41(2):216 -33.
3. McLaughlin GC. Ignore the Numbers Embrace the Data. Quality Progress. 2021;54(3).
4. Banchs RJ, Pop MR. Practicalities for Planning and Collecting Baseline Data. The Quality Improvement Challenge: A Practical Guide for Physicians. 2021;137.
5. Harsoor S, Panditrao MM, Rao S, Bajwa SJS, Sahay N, Tantry TP. Dissertation writing in post graduate medical education. Indian Journal of Anaesthesia. 2022;66(1):34.
6. Ajayi VO. Primary sources of data and secondary sources of data. Benue State University. 2017; 1(1):1-6.
7. Allen F, Steele J. Data validity and quality. Statistical and methodological aspects of oral Health Research. 2009;131-44.
8. Mays JA, Mathias PC. Measuring the rate of manual transcription error in outpatient point-of-care testing. Journal of the American Medical Informatics Association. 2019;26(3):269-72.

9. Riley J. Understanding metadata. Washington DC, United States: National Information Standards Organization (http://www niso org/ publications/press/UnderstandingMetadata pdf). 2017;23(2017):7-10.
10. Kennedy JE. Addressing researcher fraud: retrospective, real-time, and preventive strategies-including legal points and data management that prevents fraud. Front Res Metr Anal. 2024;9:1397649.
11. Patridge EF, Bardyn TP. Research electronic data capture (REDCap). Journal of the Medical Library Association: JMLA. 2018;106(1):142.
12. Little RJ, Rubin DB. Statistical analysis with missing data. John Wiley & Sons; 2019.
13. Costanzo L. Data cleaning during the research data management process. Research Data Management in the Canadian Context. 2023.
14. Schäfer RA, Voß B. RNAnue: efficient data analysis for RNA -RNA interactomics. Nucleic Acids Research. 2021;49(10):5493 -501.
15. Edemekong P, Annamaraju P, Afzal M, Haydel M. Health insurance portability and accountability act (HIPAA) compliance. StatPearls, 2024.
16. Holmes-Truscott E, Schipp J, Cooke DD, Hendrieckx C, Coates EJ, Heller SR, et al. Perceptions of adults with type 1 diabetes toward diabetes-specific quality of life measures: a survey-based qualitative exploration. Health and Quality of Life Outcomes. 2024;22(1):70.
17. Ferrante M, Ferro N, Losiouk E. How do interval scales help us with better understanding IR evaluation measures? Inf Retrieval J. 2020 Jun;23(3):289 -317.
18. Kazazis S, Depalle P, McAdams S. Interval and Ratio Scaling of Spectral Audio Descriptors. Front Psychol. 2022;13:835401.
19. Santner TJ, Duffy DE. The statistical analysis of discrete data. Springer Science & Business Media; 2012.
20. Few S, Edge P. Dual-scaled axes in graphs. Visual Business Intelligence Newsletter. 2008;1 -7.
21. Daggubati SC, Sreevalsan-Nair J, Dadhich K. Barchartanalyzer: Data extraction and summarization of bar charts from images. SN Computer Science. 2022;3(6):500.
22. Wilkinson L. How to Make a Pie. In: The Grammar of Graphics. Springer; 1999. p. 21-41.
23. Zheng B, Sadlo F. On the visualization of hierarchical multivariate data. In IEEE; 2021. p. 136-45.
24. Macdonald-Ross M. How numbers are shown: A review of research on the presentation of quantitative data in texts. AV communication review. 1977;25(4):359-409.
25. Denby L, Mallows C. Variations on the histogram. Journal of Computational and Graphical Statistics. 2009;18(1):21-31.
26. Scott DW. Frequency polygons: theory and application. Journal of the American Statistical Association. 1985;80(390):348-54.

10

CHAPTER

Dissertation Writing – The Discussion and Conclusion Sections

Ankur Khandelwal

INTRODUCTION

The discussion and conclusion sections form the crux of any dissertation, where findings are interpreted, contextualised, and synthesised in light of existing literature. This section not only highlights the significance and implications of the results but also demonstrates the researcher's critical thinking and analytical skills. The discussion should address research questions, justify interpretations, and acknowledge limitations. The conclusion then distills the key insights, outlines the study's contribution to knowledge, and suggests directions for future research. Together, these components give closure to the dissertation, reinforcing its value while situating it within the broader academic and practical framework.

DISCUSSION SECTION OF THE DISSERTATION

The discussion section of a dissertation is where postgraduate medical students synthesise their findings with existing knowledge, interpret the significance, and articulate the implications of their research. Crafting this section effectively requires a balance of critical analysis, integration of literature, and clear communication. Here are key steps and considerations for writing a compelling discussion section.[1,2]

Summarise Key Findings

Begin by succinctly summarising the main findings of your research. Avoid repeating detailed results; instead, highlight the most critical data points that answer your research questions. This sets the stage for a deeper analysis and emphasises the importance of your study.[1]

Interpret the Results

Interpretation involves explaining what the findings mean in the context of your research questions and objectives. Discuss whether your results support your hypotheses and how they compare with the existing literature. Identify patterns, relationships, and trends that emerge from your data. For example, if your research shows a significant correlation between a new treatment and patient outcomes, discuss the potential mechanisms and clinical relevance.[2,3]

Compare with Previous Research

Place your findings within the broader scientific context by comparing them with previous studies. Highlight agreements, contradictions, or extensions of prior work. This comparison can help to underscore the novelty of your research and its contribution to the field. For instance, if your findings align with previous studies, it reinforces the validity of the results. If they differ, provide possible explanations and discuss the implications of these discrepancies.[1,4]

Discuss the Implications

Detail the theoretical, clinical, and practical implications of your study. Explain how your findings advance knowledge, influence clinical practice, or suggest new avenues for research. This discussion should connect your results to real-world applications, highlighting the potential impact on patient care, medical guidelines, or future research directions.[2,5]

Acknowledge Limitations

An honest discussion of limitations is crucial for scientific integrity. Address potential weaknesses in your study, such as sample size, methodological constraints, or biases. Discuss how these limitations might affect the interpretation of your results and suggest ways to mitigate these issues in future research. This transparency enhances the credibility of your work and provides a balanced view of your findings.[2,3]

Suggest Future Research

Based on your findings and limitations, propose directions for future research. Identify gaps in knowledge that your study has highlighted and suggest specific questions that need to be addressed. This section demonstrates the ongoing relevance of your research area and encourages further investigation.

Conclude with a Strong Closing

End the discussion with a concise conclusion that reiterates the significance of your findings. Summarise the main points discussed and emphasise the overall contribution of your research to the medical field. A strong closing statement can leave a lasting impression on the reader, reinforcing the importance of your work.

Maintain Clarity and Precision

Throughout the discussion, maintain clarity and precision in your writing. Avoid jargon and overly complex sentences. Ensure that your arguments are logical and well-structured, guiding the reader through your thought process seamlessly.

Seek Feedback

Before finalising the discussion section, seek feedback from peers, mentors, or advisors. They can provide valuable insights and help identify areas that need further clarification or improvement. This iterative process can enhance the quality and rigor of your discussion.[1,4]

In summary, writing the discussion section of a dissertation involves a thoughtful integration of your findings with existing knowledge, a critical evaluation of your study's implications, and a transparent acknowledgment of its limitations. By following these guidelines, postgraduate medical students can craft a discussion that is insightful, impactful, and reflective of their contribution to the field of medicine.

STRENGTHS AND LIMITATIONS SECTION OF THE DISSERTATION

Writing the strengths and limitations of a dissertation is an important part of any research project, including a postgraduate medical dissertation. A structured approach is given in the following text.

Strengths

Methodological Rigor

- *Robust study design:* Highlight the strong design elements, such as randomised controlled trials, cohort studies, or case-control studies.
- *Comprehensive data collection:* Mention thorough and systematic data collection methods, ensuring reliability and validity.
- *Advanced analytical techniques:* If sophisticated statistical analyses or modeling techniques were used, emphasise their appropriateness and rigor.[3]

Relevance and Impact

- *Clinical relevance:* Discuss how the findings can be applied in clinical settings or influence clinical practice.

- *Public health significance:* Explain the broader impact on public health or specific patient populations.
- *Innovation:* Highlight novel aspects of the study, such as new methodologies, interventions, or findings.

Sample Size and Diversity

- *Adequate sample size:* Mention if the study had a large and statistically sufficient sample size.
- *Diverse population:* If the study includes a diverse population, explain how this enhances the generalisability of the results.

Ethical Considerations

Ethical approval: Note that the study received appropriate ethical approvals and adhered to ethical guidelines.

Sample Paragraph

"This study utilised a randomised controlled trial design, which is considered the gold standard for clinical research. The comprehensive data collection process, including regular follow-ups and objective measurements, ensured high data reliability. Additionally, the use of advanced statistical methods allowed for robust analysis of the data. The findings have significant clinical relevance, offering new insights into the management of (condition). The diverse study population enhances the generalisability of the results".

Limitations

Identify the Limitations

- *Research design:* Discuss any limitations related to your research design, such as a lack of control groups, the scope of the study, or constraints related to the research methods chosen.
- *Sample size and selection:* Mention if the sample size was small or if there were issues with sample selection that might affect the generalisability of your findings.
- *Data collection methods:* Highlight any limitations in your data collection methods, such as reliance on self-reported data, which could be biased or inaccurate.
- *Time constraints:* Explain any time limitations that might have impacted the comprehensiveness of your study.
- *Resource constraints:* Mention if limited resources (financial, human, or technical) affected your study.
- *External validity:* Discuss any factors that limit the applicability of your findings to other settings or populations.
- *Internal validity:* Acknowledge any potential biases or confounding variables that could affect the internal validity of your study.

Explain the Impact

- *Influence on results:* Describe how these limitations might have influenced the results of your study.
- *Generalisability:* Discuss how these limitations affect the extent to which your findings can be generalised to other contexts or populations.

Justify and Rationalise

- *Justification:* Provide a rationale for why certain limitations exist. For example, if the sample size was small, explain if it was due to constraints like limited access to participants or resources.
- *Rationalisation:* Discuss any steps you took to minimise the impact of these limitations, such as using robust data analysis techniques or triangulating data sources.

Discuss the Implications

- *Future research:* Suggest areas for future research that could address the limitations of your study. This shows that you recognise the need for further investigation.

- *Practical implications:* Discuss how the limitations affect the practical implications of your findings, if applicable.

Maintain a Balanced Tone

- *Objective tone:* Maintain an objective and balanced tone. Acknowledge limitations without undermining the value of your research.
- *Positive spin:* Highlight the strengths of your study and how it contributes to the existing body of knowledge despite the limitations.

Sample Paragraph

"In this study, several limitations were identified that should be acknowledged. Firstly, the sample size was relatively small, which may affect the generalisability of the findings. This limitation was due to the restricted access to participants in the study area. Additionally, the data collection method relied on self-reported questionnaires, which could introduce response bias. Despite these limitations, the study employed multiple data triangulation techniques to enhance the validity of the results. Future research could benefit from larger sample sizes and the use of objective data collection methods. Overall, while these limitations present certain constraints, the study provides valuable insights into (subject/topic), laying the groundwork for further exploration".

CONCLUSION SECTION OF THE DISSERTATION

Writing the conclusion section of a dissertation involves summarising your research findings, discussing the implications, and providing recommendations for future research and practice. A structured guide to help you write an effective conclusion is given in following text.

Restate Research Objectives

Begin by briefly restating the main objectives or research questions of your study.

Summarise Key Findings

Summarise the main findings of your research without introducing new information. Highlight the most significant results and their relevance to the research questions or hypotheses.

Discuss the Implications

- *Clinical implications:* Explain the practical implications of your findings for clinical practice. Discuss how your research can contribute to better patient care, treatment protocols, or medical guidelines.
- *Theoretical implications:* Address how your findings contribute to the existing body of medical knowledge or theories.

Acknowledge the Limitations

Briefly reiterate the limitations of your study as discussed in the limitations section. This shows transparency and a critical understanding of your research.

Recommendations for Future Research

Suggest areas for future research based on your findings and limitations. Identify specific gaps that need further investigation.

Personal Reflection (Optional)

Some dissertations may include a brief personal reflection on the research process, challenges encountered, and lessons learned. This is optional but can provide a more personal touch.

Concluding Statement

End with a strong concluding statement that encapsulates the significance of your research and its potential impact on the field of medicine.

Sample Paragraph

"In this dissertation/study, we sought to investigate the effects of (specific intervention or variable) on (specific outcome) in (specific patient population). The findings indicate that (summarise key findings), which have significant implications for clinical practice. Specifically, our results suggest that (clinical implications), thereby potentially improving patient outcomes in (specific area). However, the study is not without limitations. The sample size was relatively small, and future research should aim to include larger, more diverse populations to validate these findings. Additionally, further research is needed to explore (specific area for future research). In conclusion, this study provides valuable insights into (specific topic), contributing to the growing body of evidence supporting (specific intervention or approach). By addressing the identified gaps, future studies can build upon this work to enhance medical knowledge and practice".

CONCLUSION

In summary, the discussion and conclusion sections serve as the final and most impactful segments of the dissertation. The discussion bridges the gap between research findings and their broader significance, enabling the researcher to critically interpret results, compare them with existing literature, and reflect on their implications. A well-crafted conclusion reinforces the central arguments, acknowledges the study's limitations, and offers thoughtful recommendations for future research or practice. This chapter not only completes the research journey but also leaves a lasting impression, highlighting the scholarly contribution and relevance of the study.

REFERENCES

1. Hyatt L, Roberts CM. The Dissertation Journey: A Practical and Comprehensive Guide to Planning, Writing, and Defending Your Dissertation, 4th edition. California: Corwin Press; 2023.
2. Gastel B, Day RA. How to Write and Publish a Scientific Paper, 9th edition. California: Cambridge University Press; 2022.
3. Bui YN. How to Write a Master's Thesis, 3rd edition. Los Angeles: Sage Publications; 2019.
4. Hofmann AH. Scientific Writing and Communication: Papers, Proposals, and Presentations. 5th edition. New York: Oxford University Press; 2023.
5. Bloomberg LD. Completing Your Qualitative Dissertation: A Road Map from Beginning to End, 5th edition. California: Sage Publications; 2022.

11 CHAPTER

Academic Integrity, Copyright Issues, and Plagiarism

Mukesh Kumar Prasad, Ridhima Sharma, Rohini Dattatri, Milon V Mitragotri

INTRODUCTION

Academic integrity, copyright concerns, and plagiarism are essential for medical postgraduates involved in research, publications, and presentations. Maintaining academic honesty secures the trustworthiness of their work and aids the progress of medical knowledge. By adhering to copyright laws and steering clear of plagiarism, postgraduates protect their professional standing and avoid legal issues. Proper citation and responsible use of information are crucial for upholding the integrity of academic research.

Medical postgraduates need to comprehend the principles of academic integrity to promote the ethical sharing of knowledge, as it significantly affects the quality of medical research and patient care. Correct source attribution and compliance with copyright laws build trust and accountability within the medical profession. Support from librarians and institutions is essential in helping postgraduates address these challenges, providing them with the skills needed to prevent plagiarism.

This chapter will help to sail through the necessary knowledge and skills to navigate the complexities of academic integrity, understand copyright issues, and avoid plagiarism in research and publications. By upholding ethical principles and respecting copyright laws, the credibility of medical research and patient care can be contributed, while also protecting professional reputation from potential legal consequences.

ACADEMIC INTEGRITY

In medical education, academic integrity involves promoting a culture of learning that values intellectual honesty, critical thinking, and ethical decision-making. It entails cultivating a deep understanding of medical ethics and professional standards, as well as fostering a sense of personal responsibility for upholding these principles throughout one's career.[1]

Academic integrity demands rigorous adherence to ethical guidelines, scientific rigor, and transparency in the design, conduct, and reporting of studies in medical research. This includes obtaining informed consent from research participants, accurately collecting and analysing data, and disclosing potential conflicts of interest or sources of funding. It also warrants respecting the rights and welfare of research subjects and ensuring that research findings are reported truthfully and objectively.[1-3]

Academic integrity is defined as the commitment to uphold fundamental values in the academic community that includes:[3,4]

- Honesty
- Trust
- Fairness
- Respect
- Responsibility
- Courage

Challenges to Academic Integrity

Despite its paramount importance, academic integrity in medical colleges faces various challenges.[5,6] It includes:

- *Pressure to succeed:* Competitive nature can create pressure on students to excel academically at any cost. This pressure may tempt some students to resort to unethical behaviours such as cheating, plagiarism, or falsification of data.
- *Accessibility of resources:* In the digital age, access to online resources and study material is abundant, making it easier for students to engage in academic dishonesty by copying content or purchasing prewritten essays/ assignments.
- *Lack of awareness:* Inadequate education and awareness programmes on academic integrity may contribute to this lack of understanding.

How to make it possible?

Addressing the challenges to academic integrity in medical colleges requires a multifaceted approach that involves collaboration among educators, administrators, students, and professional organisations.[3,4,7]

Key strategies for promoting academic integrity include:

- Creating a culture of accountability.
- Education and awareness.
- Ensuring a conducive environment.
- Support services.
- Ensuring proper guidance and helping freshers to acclimatise.
- Promoting ethical role models.

Integrity Violation

Upholding academic integrity in medical colleges is essential for nurturing the next generation of competent, ethical, and compassionate healthcare professionals. By prioritising integrity in academic pursuits, medical colleges not only ensure the quality and safety of patient care but also uphold the values and reputation of the medical profession.

Integrity violation is anything that engages or attempts to engage in conduct that violates the standard of academic integrity, which could be cheating or infringement of copyright.[8]

Multiple factors may lead to violation. It could be lesser interaction among students or between students and faculty, malpractice, ghost faculty, partial behaviour, bribery, or low faculty competence.

COPYRIGHT ISSUES

What is Copyright and Copyright Exploitation?

The exclusive rights to publish and distribute a work are covered by copyright. Most countries' laws automatically grant a bundle of rights, known as "copyright", to the author or authors.[9] It combines rights against exploitation with moral rights, the most significant of which is the author's right to full and proper acknowledgment. In the system of scholarly communication, moral rights are widely recognised and maintained, even in cases where an author transfers their copyright to a publisher.

Under the conventional publishing model, the publisher typically receives all exploitation rights. This implies that reuse is restricted or reliant on the publisher's consent, which is commonly understood to mean republication and/or redistribution of the original article by a third party other than the publisher.[10] This restricts both the author's and the reader's access to the content. A collection of rights, exploitation rights represent the needs and demands of the parties concerned as well as the method of exploitation.[11] The exploitation options for research articles in scholarly communication are actually fairly limited: The two primary options are reuse for educational purposes and reuse for further research purposes.[12]

Using a Creative Commons License to Share Copyright

The open-source software movement served as some of the inspiration for the establishment of Creative Commons in 2001. Under Creative Commons, the copyright slogan "all rights reserved" has been replaced with "some rights reserved", and a number of license types have been developed to allow creators to safeguard their works while still promoting specific, approved uses. PloS and Biomed Central, two of the top publishers of open access journals, use the Creative Commons license "attribution". This license provides broad permission to use and reuse the article, including for commercial purposes, while guaranteeing the author's moral rights, namely the right to be cited through an appropriate citation. The impact of the research article on the author is maximised with this kind of license.

A prime instance of this "sharing of copyright" is found in the European Geosciences Union journals. They employ the "share alike" Creative Commons licence, which constraints reuse to open access publications.[13]

Transfer (Partly) and Copyright

Under the open access model, authors transfer all rights to commercial exploitation to the publisher but retain copyright ownership. For example, the British Medical Journal (BMJ) grants authors copyright but requires an exclusive license to publish the piece first and retains rights to commercial exploitation. The BMJ publishing group also provides authors with a portion of the royalties from any commercial republishing or redistribution agreements based on their articles.

Authors can freely use their articles without the need of permission, as long as no commercial rights are involved. They also have the opportunity to earn royalties, which is a new approach in the academic publishing field.

The postgraduate student who is the author of a dissertation, owns the copyright to his/her dissertation. The university to which the dissertation is being submitted holds a non-exclusive, royalty-free license to use and distribute the work for scholarly purposes, that means, to publish, reproduce and distribute the dissertation electronically.

In summary, copyright ensures that an author's name is always connected to their original work and prohibits publishing the same data in multiple journals without proper cross-referencing in the text and authorisation.[14,15] Revealing the same data in conference or journal notes is considered duplicate publication, which is unethical and can lead to reprimand and consequences. Redundant publication that is intentional is an unethical copyright infringement. Reprimand and discovery are possible results.[14]

How to obtain Copyright Permission for Non-original Figures/Images Used in the Dissertation?

- The copyright holder (author/publisher) of the concerned article/chapter wherein the figure originally appeared is identified.
- A mail is sent to him/her describing the proposed use of the figure.
- Written permission is obtained from the copyright holder to use the figure/image.
- It is mentioned in the dissertation that the material is reproduced with permission.

PLAGIARISM

"If you steal ideas from one author, it is plagiarism; if you steal from many, it is research".

The word plagiarism is derived from "plagiarius", a Latin word meaning "kidnapper".[16] Plagiarism is defined as "the use of others' published and unpublished ideas or words (or other intellectual property) without attribution or permission and presenting them as new and original rather than derived from an existing source" by the World Association of Medical Editors. It is a serious violation of national and international copyright laws.[17] An increasing awareness on various forms of plagiarism, editorial management, and peer review process digitalisation along with methodical scanning of multiple online platforms have enabled detection of plagiarism.[18]

Types of Plagiarism

- *Verbatim plagiarism:* This type of plagiarism occurs when the scientific matter is copied and pasted verbatim from a published article in one's own name without referencing and acknowledging the original authors. This type of plagiarism is commonly seen in the introduction and discussion part of a scientific article.[19]
- *Mosaic plagiarism:* This is a type of plagiarism wherein one's own words are added in other's opinions and ideas so that copying and pasting occur in a patchy manner.[19]
- *Paraphrasing:* This type of plagiarism occurs when a part or paragraph is rewritten in one's own words; however, it is someone else's ideas. Hence, substitution of words cannot be considered as original and can constitute plagiarism in the absence of proper referencing.
- *Cyber plagiarism:* When research articles, ideas are copied in part or entirely without proper acknowledgement of original authors, it constitutes cyber plagiarism.[19]
- *Image plagiarism:* If an image or video needs to be made use of, prior permission should be obtained, or it should be appropriately cited lest it would lead to plagiarism.[20]
- *Self-plagiarism:* Copying of one's own previously published data is considered as an act of dishonesty. It does not add to the scientific knowledge but would just help to increase the number of publications for the authors.[21] This is of four types:
  1. *Duplicate (redundant) publication:* Submitting the same article to different journals is considered duplicate (redundant) publication. This is considered as an offence, and the authors can be punished as per the Committee on Publication Ethics (COPE) flow chart.
  2. *Augmented publication:* Addition of more data to one's own previously published article, modifying the aim of the study, recalculating the results, and changing the title constitute augmented publication. This cannot be detected by the plagiarism detection software as it is not copied verbatim.
  3. *Segmented publication:* When two or more scientific papers are written from one original work, it is referred to as segmental/salami-sliced papers. It may be difficult to find out but may be pointed out by readers or manuscript reviewers.
  4. *Text recycling:* Using of a major portion of one's own published literature in the new manuscript constitutes text recycling. Plagiarism detection software can detect text recycling.

What are the major drivers of plagiarism?

The major drivers of plagiarism are enumerated in **Box 1**.[22]

Plagiarism Detection Tools

Plagiarism detection should employ both the software and human detection methods as none

BOX 1: Major causes of plagiarism.

- No awareness
- Lack of integrity
- Poor writing skills
- Publication pressure
- Deficient team culture
- Poor English language skills and cultural differences

of the currently available systems is perfect. Plagiarism detection software such as *iThenticate, Turnitin, Plagiarism.org* are popular. However, many researchers, especially in developing nations, may lack access to this proprietary software; so other freely available platforms such as Google Scholar, Grammarly, and Plagscan help to improve the acceptance rate by reputed journals.[23]

The detection of plagiarism is based on similarity scores reported by the text-matching search engines and computer software. iThenticate is the most advanced antiplagiarism tool which provides similarity score from a single source as well as overall similarity score. It has reduced but not eliminated the scientific misconduct.[24] The use of the software should not be a replacement for conscientious reading of the articles and editorial decision.

Detection of image plagiarism, an arduous task, requires the use of semantic mapping as well as processing of images.[25]

How to avoid plagiarism?

The availability of editing support, use of plagiarism detection tools before submission of manuscript, adopting institutional policies besides measures as mentioned in **Box 2** may help to avoid plagiarism.[22] Provision of a supportive environment and following high ethical standards can also help to reduce plagiarism. Guidelines such as American Medical Association (AMA) manual of style provides thorough information on scientific misconduct, ethical and legal issues, conflict of interest in addition to information regarding article preparation, punctuation, and style.[26]

BOX 2: Measures to avoid plagiarism.

- Training in research methodology
- Practice ethical writing
- Citing the sources
- Use of quotation marks when required
- Obtaining permission from the author/publisher/ copyright holder for extensive quotations and images
- Follow the editorial guidelines
- Avoid self-plagiarism
- Mastering academic English
- Avoid procrastination which leads to sloppy research and undue pressure to complete
- Improving graphic designing skills

The limits for minor, moderate, and unacceptable copying have been set by a few journals. Less than 10% copying verbatim is tolerable; 15–20% overlap of the text is less tolerable while >30% textual overlap is considered to be unacceptable.[27] However, even a small textual overlap is an ethical violation in a concealed form.

Many universities have introduced a plagiarism certification format for postgraduate dissertation. It is an undertaking that the dissertation work is an original work done by candidate, which is countersigned by the guide. The Plagiarism Check Sheet must accompany the final dissertation. It should state that plagiarism check of the content of the dissertation (except all quoted work reproduced with all necessary permissions and attribution, all references, bibliography, table of contents, preface, acknowledgements, all generic terms, laws, standard symbols and standard equations) has been done with an approved plagiarism detection tool. The percentage of similarities is mentioned in it **(Annexure 3)**. The limit of plagiarism has been set up to 10%, and if found to be above 10%, the dissertation reviewer is instructed to reject the thesis.

Citation policy should be strictly followed where 14 words are taken together from a published work, it should be cited. Where more than 40 words are copied verbatim, they should be mentioned in inverted commas ("__") in italics and needs to be cited if not from internet open sites. Contrary to this, similarity checks should exclude bibliography, acknowledgments, table of content, preface sections along with any commonly used generic words and terms.[28]

Local institutional academic committees look into all matters concerning plagiarism including decisions regarding accusations of plagiarism against faculty, students, researchers, or any staff and can decide the penalties accordingly. University level academic committees provide recommendations to local committees with regards to quantum of penalties for various offences or even repeated acts of plagiarism.[28]

Regular sensitisation programmes need to be conducted where research is commonly done to discuss the various tenets of plagiarism and its repercussions. Responsible conduct of research, publication ethics and use of plagiarism detection tools and citation tools can be discussed in these programmes.

Implications of Plagiarism

Plagiarism, an act of serious ethical offence is taken seriously by most reputed journals. The articles may be rejected during any stage of publication or may even be retracted after being published. The COPE provides guidelines for dealing with these issues.[29] The authors can be penalised, suspended, or even expelled by educational institutions, publishing companies, and professional associations for an act of copyright infringement.[19]

CONCLUSION

- In the fast-changing medical field, maintaining academic integrity is crucial. By focusing on ethical practices and honouring intellectual property rights, medical postgraduates can not only ensure excellence in their research but also enhance the integrity and trustworthiness of the medical profession.
- It is vital for medical postgraduates to grasp the implications of copyright laws when conducting research and publishing. They must be aware of the copyright status of resources, such as images, figures, and text, and ensure they follow the proper procedures for obtaining permissions and crediting the original authors accordingly.
- Plagiarism, an act of intellectual theft, is considered a serious offence in academia.
- The awareness of different prevention strategies and use of appropriate detection tools can help to avoid plagiarism.
- Using systematic search for new ideas, appropriately citing the published facts, improving the academic English and being creative in writing also help in ensuring ethical writing of the dissertation and manuscript for scientific publication.

REFERENCES

1. Morris EJ. Academic integrity: a teaching and learning approach. In: Bretag T (Ed). Handbook of Academic Integrity. Singapore: Springer; 2016. pp. 1037-53.
2. Bretag T, Mahmud S. A conceptual framework for implementing exemplary academic integrity policy in Australian higher education. In: Bretag T (Ed). Handbook of Academic Integrity. Singapore: Springer; 2016. pp. 463-80.
3. International Center for Academic Integrity. (2021). The fundamental values of academic integrity. [online] Available from https://academicintegrity.org/images/pdfs/20019_ICAI-Fundamental-Values_R12.pdf [Last accessed July, 2025].
4. Universities Australia. (2017). UA Academic Integrity Best Practice Principles. [online] Available from: https://www.universitiesaustralia.edu.au/wp-content/uploads/2019/06/UA-Academic-Integrity-Best-Practice-Principles.pdf [Last accessed July, 2025].
5. Kadayam Guruswami G, Mumtaz S, Gopakumar A, Khan E, Abdullah F, Parahoo SK. Academic integrity perceptions among health-professions' students: a cross-sectional study in the middle east. J Acad Ethics. 2023;21(2):231-49.
6. Ives B, Giukin L. Patterns and predictors of academic dishonesty in Moldovan university students. J Acad Ethics. 2020;18(1):71-88.
7. Morris EJ. Academic integrity matters: five considerations for addressing contract cheating. Int J Educ Integr. 2018;14(1):15.

8. Davis A. Academic integrity in the time of contradictions. Cogent Educ. 2023;10(2):2289307.
9. Hao M. Determination of liability for copyright infringement of online short video platforms. J Shandong Univ Sci Technol (Soc Sci Ed). 2019; 21:50-58.
10. Xiong Q. Copyright recognition of content generated by artificial intelligence. Intellectual Property. 2017;3:7.
11. Wang Q. The qualitative analysis of content generated by artificial intelligence in copyright law. Legal Sci. 2017;5:149.
12. Wang Q, Liu Y, Niu H. Exploring the status and dilemma of intellectual property subjects- from the perspective of artificial intelligence as an intellectual property subject. J Jiaozuo Univ. 2021;1:5.
13. Guo R. An analysis of the copyright subject suitability of artificial intelligence in the view of epistemology. J Beijing Inst Technol (Soc Sci Ed). 2019;4:145-54.
14. Kappel K, Luetkemeyer LM, Mannebach M. The "Rights" Prescription: Navigating Copyright Law in Practice of Medicine. Mo Med. 2024;121(4): 257-61.
15. Favre J, Germond T, Clavert P, Collin P, Michelet A, Lädermann A. Want a better h-index?—all you need to know about copyright and open access. Orthop Traumatol Surg Res. 2020;106:1475-80.
16. Aronson JK. Plagiarism - Please don't copy. Br J Clin Pharmacol. 2007;64:403-5.
17. Copyright, Designs and Patents Act 1988. [online] Available from https://www.legislation.gov.uk/ukpga/1988/48/contents [Last accessed on July, 2025].
18. Heaven D. AI peer reviewers unleashed to ease publishing grind. Nature. 2018;563:609-10.
19. Jawad F. Plagiarism and integrity in research. J Pak Med Assoc. 2013;63:1446-7.
20. Merriman J. Plagiarism - What is it? How to avoid it. Am Fam Physician 2010;82:1428.
21. Guraya SY, Guraya SS. The confounding factors leading to plagiarism in academic writing and some suggested remedies: a systematic review. J Pak Med Assoc. 2017;67:767-72.
22. Radikė M, Camm CF. Plagiarism in medical publishing: each of us can do something about it. Eur Heart J Case Rep. 2022;6(4):ytac137.
23. Magulod GC, Capulso LB, Tabiolo CDL, Luza MN, Ramada MGC. Use of technology-based tools in ensuring quality of publishable journal articles. Int J Learn Teach Educ Res. 2020;19:145-62.
24. Park S, Yang SH, Jung E, Kim YM, Baek HS, Koo YM. Similarity analysis of Korean medical literature and its association with efforts to improve research and publication ethics. J Korean Med Sci. 2017;32:887-92.
25. Eisa TAE, Salim N, Abdelmaboud A. Content-based scientific figure plagiarism detection using semantic mapping. In: Saeed F, Mohammed F, Gazem N (Eds). Emerging Trends in Intelligent Computing and Informatics. IRICT 2019. Advances in Intelligent Systems and Computing. Vol. 1073. Cham: Springer; 2020. pp. 420-7.
26. Flanagin A. Ethical and legal considerations. In: AMA Manual of Style: A guide for Authors and Editors. 11th ed. New York; 2020. pp. 171-410. Available at https://doi.org/10.1093/jama/9780190246556.003.0005. (Last accessed on Oct., 2025)
27. Kravitz R L, Feldman MD. From the Editors' Desk: Self-Plagiarism and Other Editorial Crimes and Misdemeanors. J GEN INTERN MED. 2011; 26(1). Available from https://doi.org/10.1007/s11606-010-1562-z. (Last accessed on Oct., 2025)
28. Kerala University of Health Sciences. (2018). Research: PG thesis/synopsis - PG thesis regulation [about 2 screens]. (online) Available from chrome-extension://efaidnbmnnnibpcajpcglclefindmkaj/http://www2.kuhs.ac.in/kuhs_new/images/uploads/pdf/academic/2024/PG-Thesis-Gazetted-Regulation.pdf [Last accessed on July, 2025].
29. COPE Council. COPE Flowcharts and infographics—Plagiarism in a submitted manuscript—English. Available at https://doi.org/10.24318/cope.2019.2.1(Last accessed on Oct., 2025)

12

CHAPTER

Successful Paper/Poster Presentation by Postgraduate Students

Manisha D Katikar, Sujatha MP

INTRODUCTION

Medical postgraduate students can present a paper/poster in a conference on the podium. A research paper/poster allows students to showcase their work at a scientific conference at city/state/national/international level in order to obtain instant feedback from the audience and subject experts. As per National Medical Commission rules, it is mandatory for the postgraduate student to present a minimum number of scientific papers/posters at conferences during the period of postgraduation. This also serves as a boon to the students who can present the paper at the conference, enrich their knowledge with the rich outpour of lectures at the conference, get to know their colleagues from other parts of their country, obtain an idea of the vast diversity in anaesthetic practice and exchange ideas with national and international colleagues. It increases the visibility of their research work and boosts their confidence to speak in front of professionals. The feedback received during the paper presentation can be used by the presenter to improve the paper for publication as an original research article. Nonetheless, there are many award sessions for papers and posters of postgraduate students, both at state and national conferences. The top papers/posters are selected after submission of paper abstracts and the students can present before the judges. Winning a 'best paper/poster award' can boost up the academic profile of the students which can help them in their future academic and professional life. Special points are allotted for paper presenters and award winners during recruitment interviews in medical colleges and the like. Accepted papers, especially award papers, or their abstracts are sometimes published in 'conference proceedings' which are collections of papers presented at the conference or in abstract supplements of scientific journals.

Nevertheless, it is better to do paper/poster presentation in the 2nd and 3rd year of postgraduation. The 1st year is not very suitable for this purpose, mainly because of the hectic clinical routine of the student and his/her lack of basic knowledge that makes them unable to understand the scientific deliberations that take place in a conference.

However, there is always some anxiety among the students about podium presentation as they have to present these papers in a short period of time (8–10 minutes) in front of an audience of professionals and they have to be ready to respond to the questions from the delegates. A clear and concise presentation focussing on the objectives of the paper can become a prize-winning presentation. A well-designed poster or presentation effectively highlights and communicates one's research within the academic community and produces an impact on the listeners' or reader's mind. Nevertheless, the ways to make an impactful paper/poster presentation are discussed in this chapter.

RESEARCH PAPER AND POSTER: THE DIFFERENCES AND WHICH ONE TO CHOOSE?

Both—paper and poster are powerful tools for the communication of one's research. A paper is a detailed document with a formal structure summarising original research/case reports at a conference. It is presented orally with the help of PowerPoint as a visual aid. A poster is a visual presentation of one's research findings. It is also called a 'mini-research paper' or a visual abstract. A poster is designed to be quickly understood by the viewer. It is a mixture of text, tables, graphs and photographs. It is more visually compelling and memorable than a paper. A poster can be a large piece of paper designed artistically to convey the details of the research study/case report. It can be in printed format or in electronic format. The printed format is typically displayed in a designated room/hall on poster boards/stands which are usually arranged in rows and numbered **(Fig. 1)**. The presenter has to speak about the concerned study/case report in both—paper and poster presentation before the judges. However, the time allotted for poster presentation is slightly lesser than that for a paper. Researchers/students who possess artistic talent, good-quality pictures and less superior orational skills can opt for poster presentation.

PREPARATION FOR PAPER PRESENTATION

Before beginning the preparation for the presentation, one should ask oneself the following questions:

1. What is the key message I want to convey?
2. How much time is allocated for my presentation?
3. Who is the expected audience?
4. What is the deadline and word limit for abstract submission?

Abstract: Design (Annexure 9) and Submission

The paper presentation process begins with preparation of the abstract and its submission to the scientific committee of the conference few months before the start of the conference. It is important to follow the scientific committee's guidelines, as this increases the likelihood of the paper being accepted. Adherence to the specified word limit and submission of the abstract before the deadline can maximise the chances of acceptance. Conference organisers generally prefer structured abstracts with subheadings such as Introduction, Objectives, Methodology, Results, and Conclusion. The abstract title should be catchy yet concise.

The scientific committee sends the paper abstracts to peer reviewers who select the abstracts for free paper/award paper sessions depending on the quality of the paper/poster. Nevertheless, whether it is a free paper/award paper session, questions related to the paper are asked by the judges to the presenter at the end of the presentation and there can be an interactive discussion.

Preparation of Paper

The next step is the preparation of the paper. Several important steps should be followed when starting to prepare the paper presentation:

1. The paper should be structured carefully, as a well-organised paper is always appreciated.
2. The thought process should be organised into different sections of the paper presentation.
3. An outline of the main points and their order of presentation should be created.
4. Relevant graphs, charts and photos should be included to support the presentation.
5. The key message that is to be communicated to the audience should be clearly determined.
6. Previous literature should be used to support the research question.

Parts of a Paper Presentation

Introduction: One needs to provide a brief overview of the study, outlining the purpose and background information. The introduction should clearly highlight the research question and establish the context and rationale for undertaking the study.

Aims and objectives: The overall aim of the research has to be stated and the objectives specified in clear and concise terms.

Methodology: The approach used to conduct the research including the study design, study protocol, sampling techniques and clear description of sample size determination, statistical methods planned and ethical considerations should be described.

Results: The findings of the study should be presented in a clear and organised manner. Tables, graphs or charts should be used appropriately to illustrate the data collected. A concise interpretation of the results should be provided, highlighting the key outcomes relevant to the research objectives.

Discussion: This section should offer an interpretation of the findings in the context of existing literature. It should include a comparison of the results with previous studies, discussion of the strengths and limitations and the possible practical implications of the findings of the study. A brief note on suggestions for future research directions should be added at the end.

Conclusion: The key findings should be summarised and their significance should be highlighted.

The contributors, co-workers and mentors of the study need to be acknowledged. The source of funding, if any, that made the research possible also needs to be recognised.

Visual Aids

Computer-generated presentations can be prepared using software such as Microsoft PowerPoint/Apple Keynote/Google Slides/Canva. Before beginning the preparation, it is important to be familiar with the audiovisual software that will be used during the conference. Among available options, Microsoft PowerPoint is the most widely accepted and commonly used visual aid. It is easily accessible, familiar to most people, easy to use and can support large slide sizes.

PowerPoint Presentation Structure

- It is better to avoid using fancy templates as they may distract or confuse the audience.
- Bright or loud colours should not be used.
- Overcrowding of slides with too much text should be avoided.
- It is better to avoid writing full sentences—bullet points and key phrases can be used instead.
- Visuals, diagrams and charts should be incorporated wherever possible.
- It should be ensured that slides are created in a professional style with consistent formatting.
- Clear and readable fonts such as Times New Roman should be used.
- Slides should be used to illustrate and support one's talk, and not to serve as one's script.
- Once the slides are ready, one can practise the presentation, ideally by recording himself/herself.
- The allotted time limit should always be adhered to.

Important Tips to Postgraduate Students for an Effective Presentation

- Familiarise yourself with the presentation venue and audiovisual equipment in advance.

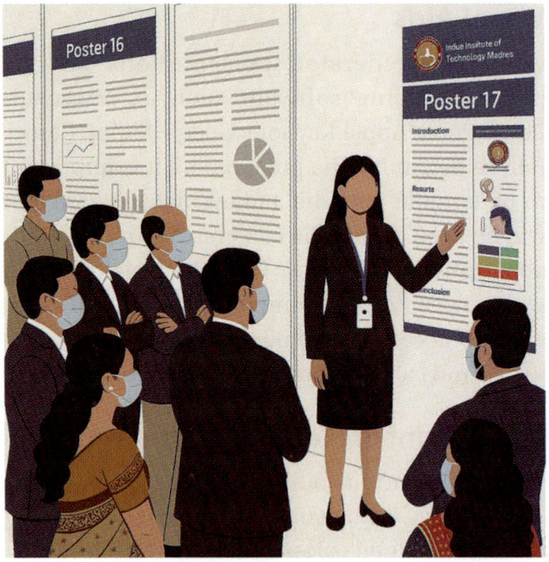

Fig. 1: Printed poster presentation.

- Begin your talk by introducing yourself (name and institution).
- Speak clearly and with a moderate pace. Avoid jargon and use simple, precise language and appropriate gestures.
- Establish eye contact with the audience and ensure your pronunciation is clear.
- Make sure to manage your time well. Finish within the allotted duration and leave time for a question-and-answer session at the end.
- Be polite and respectful while addressing questions or comments from the audience.
- Follow a formal dress code to maintain professionalism.

PREPARATION FOR POSTER PRESENTATION

Ideally a poster should have the following headings **(Annexure 10)**:

- *Title:* The title should be short, catchy and placed at the top of the poster. Names of the author and co-author, along with their affiliations, must be included. The university or conference logo with the speaker's photograph (optional) may be positioned on either side of the title.
- *Introduction or background and aim:* This consists of a brief introduction of the topic to be presented and includes the aims of the research or study with a clear research question or hypothesis.
- *Methods:* The method used in the study should be written briefly. It can be written in short sentences or in the form of a flowchart.
- *Results:* This is the heart of the poster and should include important figures, graphs and tables. This part with the key finding of the research will occupy the maximum portion of the poster.
- *Discussion:* This section should include interpreted data and explain the significance of the research.
- *Conclusions:* A few key takeaway points that convey the main message of the scientific work can be included. The research should be summarised clearly, emphasising its significance and overall contribution.
- *References:* References are to be written in the prescribed format.
- *Acknowledgements:* This can include the names of individuals who contributed to the study but did not qualify for authorship.

The abstract should not be a part of the poster.

Layout of a Poster[1]

Whenever a poster is presented at a conference, the guidelines provided by the organisers with respect to the poster size and general layout need to be followed. Microsoft PowerPoint and Canva are user-friendly, online graphic design tools that can be used to make high quality and high impact posters. Sometimes, organisers might supply poster templates with logos and colour schemes. If no template is provided, a customised poster design should be selected.

The information in a poster should flow from top to bottom and left to right. Numbers

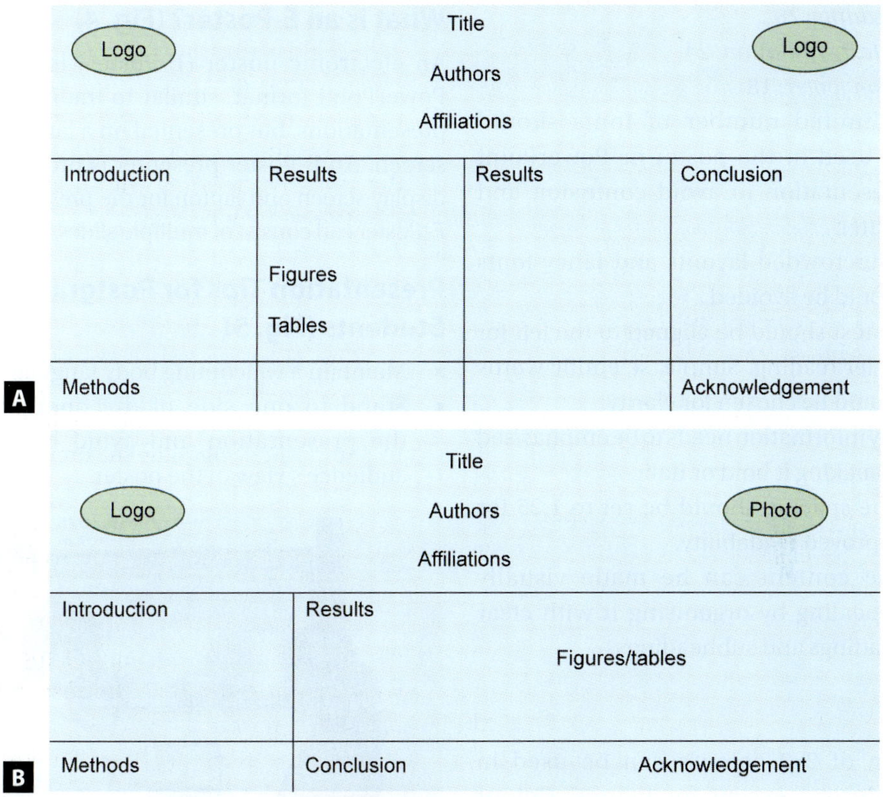

Figs. 2A and B: Landscape layout.[1]

or arrows can be used to indicate the sequence of information. Posters can be formatted in landscape or portrait layout **(Figs. 2 and 3)**.

In the landscape layout, the poster is divided into 2–4 columns. Maximum portion (1–2 columns) of the poster is used for the results. Text should not be too long and should have narrow width. The allocation of poster space is: Text: 20–25%, Figures/Tables: 40% and Empty/Free Space: 40%.

- *Formatting:* Short bullet points can be used in the poster instead of paragraphs. A clear, readable font such as Arial or Sans Serif can be selected.
- *Text font size:* Should be readable from a distance of 5 feet. The recommended font size is as follows—
  - *Title:* 72–80
  - *Heading:* 36–48

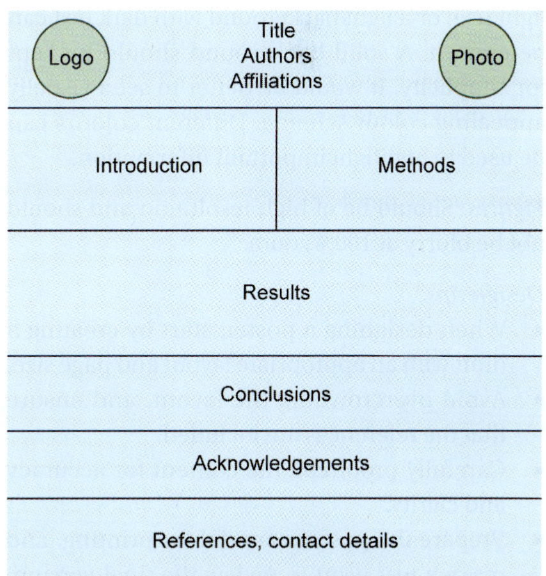

Fig. 3: Portrait layout.[1]

- *Subheading:* 28
- *Body text, affiliation:* 24
- *Caption footer:* 18
    - A limited number of fonts should be used in the poster or PowerPoint presentation to avoid confusion and clutter.
    - Overcrowded layouts and fancy fonts should be avoided.
    - All text should be aligned to the left for easier reading. Simple, scientific words should be chosen for clarity.
    - Key information needs to be emphasised by making it bold or italic.
    - Line spacing should be set to 1.25 for improved readability.
    - The content can be made visually appealing by organising it with clear headings and subheadings.

Colours

A maximum of 2–3 colours can be used in the poster design, except for figures. Colour combinations such as a dark background with light text, or a light background with dark text can be chosen. A solid background should be kept for simplicity. It would be better to set a visually appealing colour scheme. Different colours can be used to highlight important information.

Figures: Should be of high resolution and should not be blurry at 100% zoom.

Design tips:

- When designing a poster, start by creating a draft with an appropriate layout and page size.
- Avoid overcrowding the layout, and ensure that the references are included.
- Carefully proofread the content for accuracy and clarity.
- Prepare the poster material for printing, and make a test print to review the final version. For best results, print your poster on glossy, semi-glossy paper or foldable flex material.

What is an E-Poster? (Fig. 4)

An electronic poster (E-Poster) is a poster in PowerPoint format, similar to traditional poster presentations, but presented on a large computer screen. An E-Poster presenter is provided with a display screen and laptop for the presentation. The E-Poster can consist of multiple slides/just one slide.

Presentation Tips for Postgraduate Students (Fig. 5)

- Maintain a welcoming body language.
- Stand to one side of the podium during the presentation and avoid blocking the audience's view of the poster.

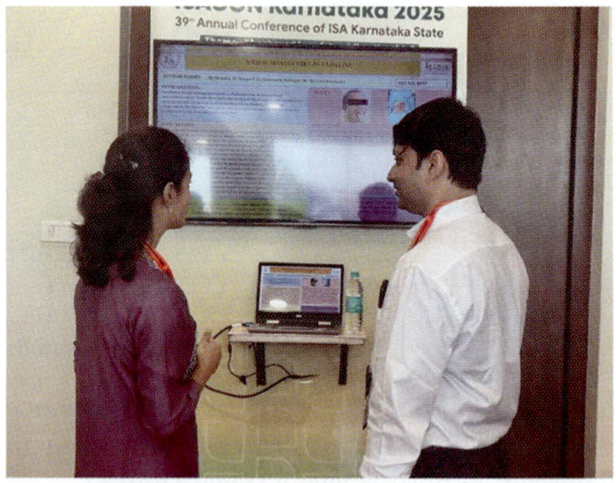

Fig. 4: An electronic poster.

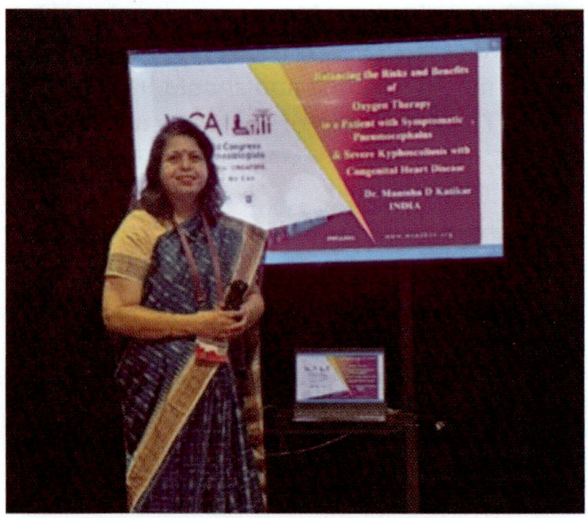

Fig. 5: The author of this chapter presenting a poster.

- Give a brief outline of the problem, approach, major findings, conclusions and significance of your work.
- Use a pointer to highlight relevant parts of the poster.
- Look at the audience, not the poster.
- Deliver the presentation within the scheduled time.
- Speak at a normal pace, focussing on important points only.
- Emphasise key points by changing your tone and pace.
- Use simple language.
- Make eye contact with all listeners.
- Make imaginative use of captioned illustrations and photographs.
- *For E-poster:*[2]
    - Be clear and concise.
    - Avoid overcrowding.
    - Use fonts that are large enough to read at a distance.
    - Put light-coloured fonts on dark backgrounds or vice versa.
    - Add high-quality graphics and videos; sound may not be permitted in some places.
    - Avoid hyperlinks. Incorporate a Quick Response (QR) code into your presentation that contains more information about your research.
    - Single slide/multiple slide presentation templates with sample layout may be provided by the organisers. Use these for preparing your poster.

CONCLUSION

Successful paper and poster presentations increase the visibility of academic work. The interactions with colleagues and organising committee professionals help in the development of communication skills. The entire process boosts the postgraduate student's confidence in presenting academic work before professionals. This can enable the overall academic growth of the postgraduate student.

REFERENCES

1. Xplorebio. Research and Publishing Series. How to make a great research poster? Academic poster design for conference (Phd). Layout and formatting. Online video clip. [online] Available from https://www.youtube.com/watch?v=5TBs2SL6LLc&t=298s. [Last accessed August, 2025]
2. QDET-2. E-Poster Presentation Tips. [online] Available from https://ww2.amstat.org/meetings/qdet2/presentationtips.cfm. [Last accessed in August, 2025]

13 CHAPTER

Strategies for Successful Completion of a Dissertation

Jagadish G Sutagatti, Madhuri S Kurdi, Ullasa Lingaraju

"The only source of knowledge is experience".
—Albert Einstein

INTRODUCTION

Dissertation writing is a collaborative effort between the student and the postgraduate (PG) guide. Its successful completion involves various aspects such as fundamental knowledge of research and dissertation writing, teacher-student sincerity, a good teacher-student relationship, approach to the co-guide, communication skills of the teacher and the student, and the reaction of the guide and student during difficult times.

BASIC KNOWLEDGE OF RESEARCH AND DISSERTATION WRITING

Poor knowledge of research methodology and lack of knowledge regarding recent advances in the subject can lead to the formation of a "not-so novel" research hypothesis, an incorrect or weak study design, incorrectly framed titles, unclear objectives, non/incorrect estimation of sample size at the beginning of the study, incorrect application of statistical tests, and poor representation of collected data. Nevertheless, when a PG student begins their course, they are usually new to research and thesis writing. However, some students may have prior exposure to research through undergraduate courses, such as the Indian Council of Medical Research (ICMR) research projects and those conducted in the Department of Preventive and Social Medicine. There are also various biomedical research courses offered by universities and institutions, such as the Basic Course in Biomedical Research (BCBR) examination conducted by the National Institute of Epidemiology (NIE) and the ICMR. Research methodology workshops organised at national conferences are another valuable source of learning. In many medical colleges, the Department of Preventive and Social Medicine organises a one day workshop on the basics of research for newly joined PG students. For PG teachers, all faculty members must clear the BCBR examination conducted by the NIE and ICMR to become eligible for faculty promotions in medical colleges. Some PG guides gain experience by co-guiding students from other departments. Younger PG guides observe the guidance provided by senior guides and learn from their experiences. As the old saying goes, "*The first time you do something is always exciting*", and for PG guides, their own experiences as students while writing dissertations are valuable sources of learning. Once a teacher begins guiding students, there is no turning back—the experience of guiding each student is unique, and the lessons learned accumulate over time. Journal clubs, which are part of the PG curriculum, contribute significantly to students' understanding of scientific and research methodologies.

TEACHER-STUDENT SINCERITY

Sincerity is essential on both sides throughout the research and dissertation writing process. It is particularly important at stages such as formulating the research hypothesis, writing the synopsis, conducting the research, collecting data, and performing statistical analysis. A casual approach at any of these stages can lead to an incomplete or non-novel thesis, errors in data collection, data fabrication, unethical practices, and unreliable conclusions. The PG student must be diligent, sincere, and meticulous in conducting their research. Insincerity often becomes apparent when the dissertation is examined by external examiners or when the thesis is later turned into an article for journal publication and gets rejected.

POSTGRADUATE GUIDE-STUDENT RELATIONSHIP (FIG. 1)

A student looks to their guide for knowledge, guidance, and skill acquisition, while the guide expects the student to be honest, sincere, and innovative in their research approach. The most significant interaction between the PG guide and the student occurs during the formulation of the research hypothesis, writing the synopsis, meeting with the ethical committee, statistical analysis, and analysing the study's results. Finally, the dissertation writing process is where their relationship culminates. Teachers and students may have different personalities, but their bond strengthens as time progresses. During the search for a research hypothesis, the PG student is often like a newborn baby in the hands of their mother—unsure of what to do. It is essential for PG students to interact frequently with their guide, updating them on progress and discussing any challenges encountered during the research. In turn, the guide's motivation, support, and enthusiasm help the student stay focused and continue collecting data despite a busy clinical routine. An impatient or egoistic teacher can create bitterness in their students, while a teacher's humility and patience develop over time and with experience. A sincere student with novel ideas will inspire encouragement in the mind of the PG guide, further enriching their relationship.

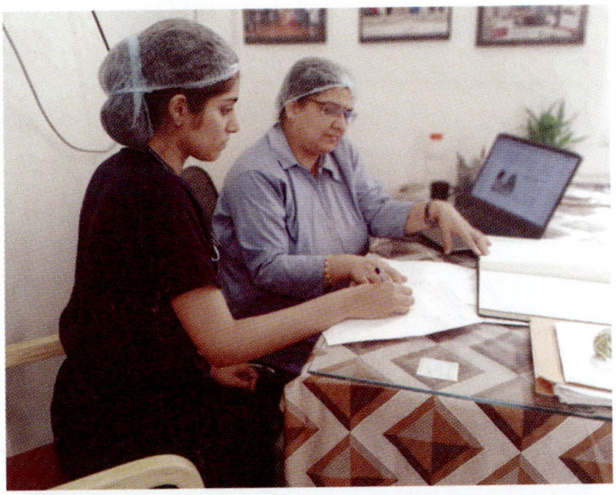

Fig. 1: Postgraduate teacher-student interaction. (The author of this chapter interacting with her student)

APPROACH TO THE CO-GUIDE

Some dissertations require a co-guide. For example, a thesis on obstetric patients may need an obstetrician as a co-guide. The relationship with the co-guide is also crucial. The PG student must make time to consult the co-guide and keep them informed about the research's progress. Humility, effective time management, and sincerity play an essential role in gaining the guidance, support, and cooperation of the co-guide.

COMMUNICATION SKILLS BETWEEN TEACHER AND STUDENT

Effective communication is vital in all areas of life, and dissertation writing is no exception. Good communication between the teacher and student can prevent misunderstandings, build trust, and avoid errors in the research process. It fosters a positive and research-friendly environment, reducing mental exhaustion and feelings of boredom. Warnings or suggestions from the teacher should be taken seriously by the student, and appropriate actions should be taken to ensure the successful conduct of the research.

TIME MANAGEMENT

One of the most critical aspects of successful dissertation completion is effective time management. It is easy for students to become overwhelmed by their responsibilities, especially when balancing clinical work, classes, and dissertation research. Setting realistic goals and adhering to a structured timeline helps keep students on track. Breaking the dissertation process into smaller, manageable tasks and setting deadlines for each can help prevent procrastination. Regularly revisiting and adjusting the timeline as needed ensure steady progress. The head of the department and the PG guide regularly assess the progress of the research work and dissertation writing.

ADAPTING TO CHANGES AND IMBIBING NEWER INFORMATION

Research is not a linear process. As new information emerges or obstacles arise, the student may have to modify the methodology. In such a situation, the reapproval of the modified methodology by the hospital ethics committee is necessary. Also, the modification has to be informed in time to the concerned university and the Clinical Trials Registry-India.

MAINTENANCE OF COMPOSURE AND PATIENCE IN ADVERSE CIRCUMSTANCES

Sometimes, the dissertation process will be marred by unhappy moments such as rejection/major revision of the synopsis, shortage/failure of equipment and devices needed to conduct the study, failure to complete/submit the dissertation in time due to the cropping up of personal or technical problems, and finally, rejection of the dissertation. At such times, the guide and student need to remain calm and composed. Nonetheless, they should analyse their mistakes, work out on the lacunae, make the necessary corrections, and move forward. Frustration at any juncture is unwarranted.

CONCLUSION

Dissertation writing requires sincerity, innovative ideas, and collaboration between the guide and the student. A strong teacher-student relationship strengthens the research process and paves the way for quality research and the development of future PG teachers. A lapse in effort from either side can lead to flaws in the thesis and, ultimately, a lifetime of regret.

14 CHAPTER

Examination of a Dissertation

Geeta Singariya, Parul Jindal, HG Manjunath

INTRODUCTION

Dissertation is a compulsory part of the 3-year postgraduate (PG) academic curriculum for obtaining a degree (e.g., master's and PhD). Examination of a dissertation is the process in which the student's research work is reviewed, critiqued, and assessed for its quality, originality, and contribution to the field according to academic standards. Most universities give a set of instructions and guidelines about their expectations from the candidates much in advance.

KEY ELEMENTS IN A DISSERTATION

A dissertation should contain new scientific knowledge, demonstrate critical thinking on the candidate's part, familiarity with the field, scientific integrity and adhere to the ethical norms of research. The dissertation should have the following key elements:

- *Originality:* The research should be original and make a significant contribution to the field. The idea of research should be as novel as possible. The chances of a thesis or paper being published in the future depends on the novelty of the research topic.
- *Depth of research:* Examiners will assess the depth and breadth of the research conducted, including the research question, literature review, methodology, analysis, and conclusion. The thesis should mention the various research methods used; the various formulas applied as well as the various statistical methods used.
- *Coherence and organisation:* A well-structured and written thesis is important, as it demonstrates the ability to communicate complex ideas effectively. To create a coherent thesis, the student might organise and write as per the typical structure of other theses and journal articles in the field. This would also help the candidate and the examiner to steer the viva on the thesis in a definitive direction without any confusion.
- *Critical analysis:* Examiners expect to see evidence of critical thinking and analysis throughout the thesis, including the ability to evaluate and interpret data and literature.
- *Contribution to knowledge:* The thesis should demonstrate how it adds to the existing body of knowledge in the field. A thesis could be a continuation or a modification to evaluate the results of an older study, but the idea should add to the existing study and amplify its worth. Thesis examiners tend to be broadly consistent in their practices and recommendations. As academic readers, they favour a thesis that engages with the literature review (comprehensive and up to date), has a convincing approach, analyses the findings, and is publishable. In fact, being publishable and making a contribution to the literature is the most important thing examiners look for.

- *Rigor and validity:* Examiners will assess the rigor of the research methods and the validity of the findings. Here, the idea of plagiarism comes into account. With the advent of the availability of tonnes of articles and data on the net, the incidences of plagiarism have emerged increasingly.
- *Clarity and style:* A well-written thesis with clear and concise language is important for effective communication of ideas. Repetitions should be minimum, and points should be put across as extremely short and crisp. Lengthy paragraphs should be avoided.
- Overall, examiners are looking for a high-quality piece of original research that demonstrates the candidate's ability to engage with complex ideas and contribute meaningfully to their field of study.

NATIONAL MEDICAL COMMISSION GUIDELINE REGARDING DISSERTATION/THESIS

The National Medical Commission (NMC) has released a notification that has proposed certain changes in the postgraduate medical education curriculum, regarding dissertation/thesis (Regulation 8.4 of the Post Graduate Medical Education Regulations 2023). Accordingly, the thesis will be a part of the clinical/practical examination and *"5% marks (20 marks) of total marks in the clinical/practical and viva voce components will be of dissertation/thesis".* By incorporating the thesis viva into the practical examination, the NMC aims to ensure that students not only possess theoretical knowledge but also practical skills in research, which are crucial for their future careers as medical practitioners and researchers. The addition of a thesis viva to the practical examination for postgraduate medical education is aimed at enhancing the assessment of both research and communication skills and encouraging students to develop their ability to discuss complex medical concepts clearly and confidently, an essential skill for any healthcare professional.

The dissertation/thesis will be evaluated by an external examiner from outside the state, who will also conduct the viva voce on it including questions related to the research study that has been conducted. Marks will be awarded as per the quality of dissertation/thesis **(Table 1, Annexure 11)** and performance in the viva voce.

Which parts of the thesis do examiners tend to read in depth? What questions on dissertation can be asked in the PG exams?

A good dissertation should be presented under the following headings: Title, abstract, introduction, aim and objectives of the study, description of devices if any or pharmacology of drugs, review of literature, materials and methods, sample size, statistical analysis, observations and results, discussion, conclusions, limitations of the study, references, study proforma, and master chart.

Thesis examiners, being time-constrained, often focus on specific sections of a thesis. Although some sections are read more closely, the examiner will review the entire thesis to make sure it is in good shape and nothing important is missed. While the entire thesis is technically evaluated, certain parts focus more in-depth scrutiny. The key areas include:

- *Abstract:* The abstract serves as a concise summary of the entire thesis and gives a brief overview of the research. A well-written abstract sets a positive first impression and provides a roadmap for the examiner. If the abstract is poorly written, the examiner might be less inclined to read the rest of the thesis in detail.
- *Introduction:* The introduction sets up the research question and provides context. Examiners scrutinise this section to assess the clarity of the research objectives, problem statement, and rationale for the study.

TABLE 1: Dissertation evaluation sheet.

S. No.	*Heading*	*Evaluation items*
1	Title	Have the FINER criteria, the acronym for feasibility, topical interest, novelty, ethicality, and relevance been used to create the research topic? The PICOT method, which describes the patient, intervention, comparison, outcome, and time, would help to generate a specific and well-formulated research question.
2	Abstract	Does the abstract contain rationale for the study, hypothesis and objectives, methods, major findings, and conclusion?
3	Introduction	Does the student present enough and relevant background/rationale on what is known about the topic, existing information gap, and importance of bridging that gap? Is the research question clearly defined, focused, and significant? Does the introduction provide sufficient context to understand the research?
4	Aim and objectives	Are the aims of the study, primary and secondary objectives, clearly stated and aligned with the research question?
5	Review of literature	Does the student cite enough relevant literature properly to support the information presented and answer the research question, hypothesis, and objectives? Does the student synthesise the literature to identify gaps, contradictions, and opportunities for the research?
6	Materials and methods	Is there enough detail of what, when, where, and how the research was performed so that the other researcher can repeat the method for similar studies? (Details about the study design, setting, locations, and relevant dates, including periods of recruitment, exposure, follow-up, and data collection should be included in the thesis) What are the eligibility criteria and methods of case ascertainment and control selection? What method is used for randomisation, group allocation, and blinding? Are the primary and secondary outcome measures completely defined? How and when were they assessed?
7	Sample size	Is the method of sample size estimation mentioned?
8	Statistical analysis	Are the appropriate statistical tests used and interpreted correctly? What statistical methods are used to compare groups for primary and secondary outcomes? What methods were used to examine subgroups and interactions and how missing data were addressed?
9	CONSORT diagram	Is the CONSORT diagram presented if it is a randomised controlled trial?
10	Results	Are the key results presented clearly, logically, accurately, and effectively (e.g., using tables and figures)? Are the findings presented objectively in relation to the research question and objectives?
11	Discussion	Does the author interpret the findings correctly and in relation to the literature? Does the author discuss the implications of the findings for the field of study?
12	Conclusion	Does the conclusion satisfy the problems being stated on the paper?
13	Limitations	Does the author acknowledge the limitations of the research, taking into account sources of potential bias or imprecision? Are suggestions for future research appropriate and insightful?
14	References	Are the references properly cited? Are they complete? What is the quality of the sources used?
15	Study proforma	It should be a blueprint document that details the key aspects of the research process in a way that helps with the planning, organisation, and tracking progress. It should emphasise the practical aspects and steps involved in the research.
16	Master chart	It should be a visual representation of the entire research structure, outlining the key components, sections, and their interconnections. It should contain all the demographic details of the patients, objectives of the study, and tabulation (variables)—systematic arrangement of classified data.

(CONSORT: Consolidated Standards of Reporting Trials)

- *Literature review:* This section demonstrates the student's understanding of the existing body of knowledge. Examiners will carefully review how well the research is formulated within the field, research gaps are identified, and the study's contribution to the field.
- *Methodology:* A key place where examiners focus their licensing attention is on the chapter that outlines the design and conduct of the research. The "methods" chapter, as it is often called and as it appears in the thesis, is not a mindless ritual, something to be done just because it has to be written. It is the place where the student demonstrates the knowledge of how to design and conduct research—not just this one project, but others in the future. There are three things that most examiners look for in a methods chapter. They look at: Research design, data generation, and data analysis.[1]
- *Results:* While this section is often more straightforward, examiners will still look carefully at how the data are presented and what statistical tests are used. They want to see clear, precise findings that align with the research questions.
- *Discussion:* This section is critical, as it shows how well the student has interpreted the results and placed them within the context of the existing literature. Examiners will closely read this part to assess the student's ability to critically analyse the data and contribute to the field with new insights. They will check whether the strengths and limitations of the study are mentioned.
- *Conclusion:* Examiners focus on how well the research is summarised and reflect on its implications. They also check if practical or theoretical implications of the conducted research and avenues for future research are suggested.

Examiners often apply Glassick's criteria for assessing the quality of scholarship of a research study. These criteria include

- *Clear purpose:* Goal/research question and supporting rationale.
- *Adequate preparation:* Thorough, integrated review of relevant literature and prior work.
- *Use of appropriate research approach and methods:* To answer the research question.
- *Effective presentation:* In a way that others can emulate and build upon.
- *Reflective critique:* Regular systematic approach to the question and learning from the research process.[2]

Throughout the thesis, examiners may also check for consistency in the arguments, logical flow, clarity, and accuracy in sentence formation including grammar.

Some secrets about examination of a thesis:

- Most examiners judge the thesis by the end of the third chapter itself. So, one has to make sure that the beginning of the thesis is impressive. The approach to a thesis should be convincing from the very beginning for the examiner to be able to stay hooked to it till the end. Spelling mistakes, especially in the title, irritate the examiners and put them off.
- Examiners are mostly consistent in their ways of assessment and mostly pass the thesis with minor revisions **(Annexure 11)**. Rarely, examiners might reject a dissertation for failure to choose a contemporary topic, a poor review of literature, defective methodology, biased analysis, or incorrect conclusions.[3]
- Most examiners enjoy the process of reading the thesis. The thesis should make a good read.
- Thesis examiners make judgments about the quality of a thesis and also offer constructive, formative feedback about how to improve.[4]

CONCLUSION

A good dissertation reflects a carefully executed study, presented clearly under key sections such as structure, methods, analysis, evidence, and originality. The review of such a dissertation reveals that the research was carried out in a thoughtful and organised manner. The dissertation is evaluated to find out whether the candidate has shown a solid grasp of the research question and has successfully placed the study within the correct theoretical and practical frameworks. Overall, the evaluation should confirm that the dissertation has the potential to offer valuable insights and contribute meaningfully to the concerned academic discipline.

REFERENCES

1. Harsoor SS, Panditrao MM, Rao S, Bajwa SJS, Sahay N, Tantry TP. Dissertation writing in post graduate medical education. Indian J Anaesth. 2022;66(1):34-46.
2. Johnson JL, Adkins D, Chauvin S. A review of the quality indicators of rigor in qualitative research. Am J Pharm Educ. 2020;84(1):7120.
3. Patter. (2017). Three things examiners look for in methods chapters. [online] Available from https://patthomson.net/2017/06/26/three-things-examiners-look-for-in-methods-chapters [Last accessed July, 2025].
4. Golding C. Advice for writing a thesis (based on what examiners do). Open Rev Educ Res. 2017;4(1):46-60.

15

CHAPTER

Successful Scientific Publication by Postgraduate Students

Sukhminder Jit Singh Bajwa, Madhuri S Kurdi

"Reading maketh a full man, conference a ready man, but writing an exact man".

—Francis Bacon

"Work, finish and publish".

—Michael Faraday

INTRODUCTION

The dissertation provides the first exposure to scientific research for any postgraduate (PG) student. Once the dissertation is completed, it is time to exhibit the research to a larger audience in the form of a paper or poster at a conference or as an article in a scientific journal. The dissertation is usually accepted by the university before the student appears for his/her PG examinations. Once it is presented and accepted by the university, the study can be published in a scientific journal. The journal clubs are a mandatory part of the PG curriculum, and they play an important role in introducing the world of scientific publications to the PG student. Understanding and following clinical practice guidelines published by the authorised bodies is an important part of PG training, and these guidelines are published in the speciality journals. The search for these published guidelines orients the students toward scientific journals. A visit to the institute library can demonstrate the several hundreds of medical journals, and this can attract medical students to the world of publications.

Why publish?

The National Medical Commission in our nation mandates that a minimum number of publications are necessary for PG students and for faculty recruitment and promotions in medical colleges.[1] A dissertation once published as an original article can become an asset, both for the student trying to get a job in medical colleges as faculty and for the PG guide who will be trying for faculty promotion in the department. Nevertheless, scientific publishing helps to improve networking within the scientific community and helps to improve the curriculum vitae of the author. Publication is an important part of a person's academic career. The academic ranking of an institute depends a lot on the publication output of its faculty and students.

What and how to publish?

The thesis can be published as an article in a medical journal. The PG student and teacher conduct the study and write the article together, and this can be done after the student clears his/her PG examination. Nonetheless, the research study of the dissertation can be presented by the student as a paper or poster at a conference initially and later on published as an article in a scientific journal. This is very useful because the lacunae in the study are often questioned by the audience during the paper presentation, and these can be corrected when the paper is submitted to a journal for publication.

Publications can be in various categories or of different types. The research in the form of a randomised controlled trial (RCT)/case control study/cohort study/retrospective study can be published as an original article/clinical communication/letter to the editor (correspondence). Further, there are other article categories that can be of interest to PG students such as case series/technical reports/pictorial essays/case reports.[2,3] A student often encounters difficult/rare cases/unusual clinical observations during the period of postgraduation. These can be published as case reports/letter to editor. Nevertheless, original research articles, especially RCTs, occupy a high position in the hierarchy of evidence **(Fig. 1)**.[4]

More than five clinical cases with same presentation or observation can be published as a case series. Case series is a type of observational or descriptive study that follows a group of patients who have a similar diagnosis or who are undergoing the same procedure over a certain period of time. Case series serve as a means of initially reporting on novel diagnostic or therapeutic strategies. The purpose of a case series should be the generation of a hypothesis, which subsequently can be tested in studies of greater methodological rigor. A case series will not have a control group and may be prospective or retrospective. Data are not measured in a standardised way, and a case series is prone

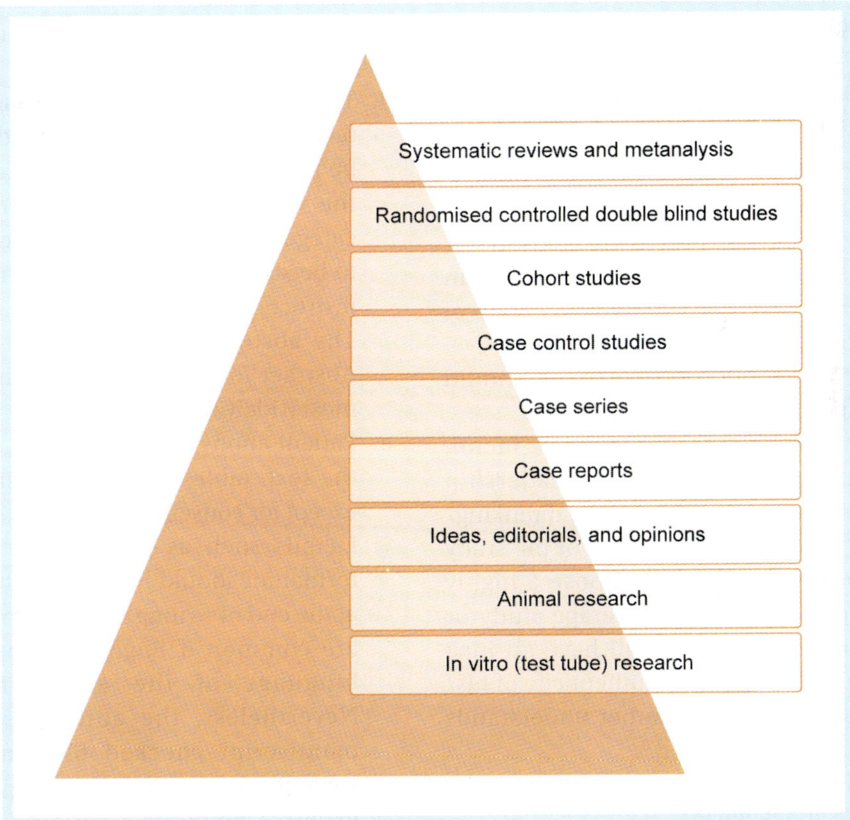

Fig. 1: Pyramid of evidence-based medicine.

to bias. A case series is lower than a RCT in the hierarchy of evidence but is useful when a RCT is not possible. It can save a lot of time and money when compared to a RCT.[4] The ideal case series has a prospective design, has an institutional ethics committee approval, and contains a clear definition of its population, intervention, outcomes, and amount of follow-up.

A technical report is a short report about a procedure/technique that is new or a technical experience of the author that is of interest to the reader.

Pictorial essays are descriptive essays on a subject. They are well illustrated with a large number of figures and are useful as a teaching modality. Technical reports and pictorial essays are accepted in surgery-related journals and journals of radiodiagnosis.

STEPS AND TIPS FOR WRITING A MANUSCRIPT FOR PUBLICATION

"Manuscript" means the article or written presentation that is submitted to a journal.

1. The right journal has to be chosen for submitting the manuscript. One has to log in to the journal website and find out details of the journal such as:
    a. Is it a predatory journal? One should avoid submitting to such journals.
    b. The journal indexing, impact factor, article rejection rate, and readership should be checked. The journal ranking/level should suit the quality of the study or article. One cannot choose a highly ranked journal for an average study or article. Every author will have an idea about the quality and authenticity of his/her study just as a mother understands the caliber of her child.[2]
    c. The journal should suit the subject of the article and language.
    d. Details of the peer review process and time for publication of articles in the chosen journal should be looked for. If in a hurry to publish, one has to go for journals with fast-track peer review process. However, all standard journals require a minimum of 3 months (average 3–6 months) from submission to publication. There can be a long waiting period of 1–2 years in some journals.
    e. One has to check whether it is an open access journal. Some journals publish articles free of cost. Some waive off fees in part or whole.
2. The author instructions for the chosen journal should be read in detail.
3. One has to decide what category of article the concerned research (of the thesis) fits in. For example, original article/clinical communication/case report/case series/letter to the editor.
4. The proper format of headings has to be followed, and appropriate headings should be used as per the category of article. Also, the word count permitted for the article category and the number of references is to be strictly followed as per journal author instructions **(Table 1)**.
5. The abstract is to be written in the last. Abstract forms the heart of the article, is most widely read and should be well written.
6. Patient anonymity has to be maintained in the text, tables, figures, and photographs except for consent form.
7. Details such as grammar and sentence formation should be checked meticulously at the end of writing.[3] Grammatical mistakes are common if English is not the native language of the author/researcher. Nevertheless, the authors can get the manuscript checked for grammar and sentence formation by an English language expert. Commercial services for English language editing are also available and are aligned to several journals.[5,6]

TABLE 1: Headings for different article categories.

Type of article	***Headings***
Original article	• *Title* • *Abstract:* Structured (background and objective, methodology, results, and conclusion) • *Keywords:* Usually 3–10 medical subject heading (MeSH) words preferably • *Article proper:* IMRaD pattern – I: Introduction (What question was asked?) – M: Methodology (How was it studied?) – R: Results (What was found?) – a: and – D: Discussion (What do the findings mean?) • *Conclusion* • *References:* 25–30; usually Vancouver style followed for citation, but there can be other styles • *Acknowledgement:* For those who helped but do not qualify to be authors • *Figures and tables:* As per rules of the journal, usually 4–6 in number with legends to be mentioned below the table • Word count permitted: Usually 2,500–3,000 words (minus the abstract and references) Abstract: 250 words • Follow Consolidated Standards for Reporting (CONSORT) guidelines when original article is based on an RCT • Follow Strengthening the Reporting of Observational Studies (STROBE) guidelines when original article is an observational study
Case report	• *Title* • *Abstract:* Unstructured • *Keywords* • *Introduction* • *Case report* • *Discussion* • *Conclusion* • *References* • Word count permitted: Approximately 800 words (minus abstract and reference) Abstract: 150 words • Follow CARE case report guidelines while writing
Case series	• *Title* • *Abstract:* Unstructured • *I: Introduction* (What question was asked?) • *M: Methodology* (How was it studied?) • *R: Results* (What was found?) • *D: Discussion* (What do the findings mean?) (for formal case series) • Introduction, case description, discussion, conclusion (for informal case series) • *Conclusion* • *References*
Letter to editor	• No abstract or keywords • *Title* • Start the letter as *Sir/Dear Editor,* • *Body* • Word count: Approximately 500 words (minus references)

8. The style of reference citation, and number and style of tables and figures should be strictly followed as per journal author instructions.
9. Numerical data, figures, and tables should be checked multiple times for accuracy. Several journal editors ask to see raw data, and one has to preserve the data for at least 5 years.
10. After manuscript submission, one has to show patience. The editorial team initially goes through the manuscript; the manuscript undergoes peer review (single/double blinded/open). Peer reviewers are experts in the subject who go through the manuscript, find out the authenticity of the study, check the data, statistics, and the way the manuscript is written. They give their critical comments and suggestions to the authors and editor to improve the article. The comments are sent to the author, and the author revises the article and resubmits it. This process goes on till the reviewers and editors are satisfied. The rejection/acceptance of the manuscript depends on the final recommendation of the reviewers to the editor.
11. The article if rejected can be submitted to another journal where it may be accepted. Some journals even suggest the names of journals to which the article can be resubmitted. One should never lose heart. There is always a place for every article. Nevertheless, the authors can share their unpublished studies on preprint servers. Preprint servers are repositories that contain data or work related to different scholarly papers that are not yet peer-reviewed or accepted by the academic journals. Authors can receive early feedback on their articles that are shared on preprint servers.

    Common reasons for manuscript rejection:[2,3]
    i. Lack of necessary skills and experience in writing
    ii. Poor research design: Poorly planned, conducted, and presented research
    iii. Errors in statistical techniques
    iv. Lack of novelty in research
    v. Grammatical errors
    vi. Selection of incorrect journal for publication
    vii. Author misconduct including plagiarism
12. The manuscript should never be simultaneously submitted to more than one journal. It should be resubmitted to another journal only after getting a decision from the journal editorial team. Plagiarism is a commonly observed form of author misconduct, which should be avoided. The manuscript should be screened for plagiarism and the similarity score on iThenticate/Turnitin/other software should be obtained before manuscript submission. Most journals will have a maximum similarity score of 3–10%, beyond which the article will not be accepted.

    One should keep away from scientific fraud because it is easily detectable and when detected can easily end the academic career of the author.
13. Some PG students often forget to put their PG guide's name as first/second author in the paper/poster/publication. There are unfortunate instances of PG students having forgotten/purposefully not put their PG guides name as author. This is unforgivable.
14. One should remember that writing a scientific paper is both an art and a science. It requires patience and firm determination to get one's research work published.

CONCLUSION

PG students have a lot of opportunities to publish in scientific journals. The research of the PG dissertation is an ideal resource to publish, and it is usually the PG student's first scientific publication. Besides the thesis, there are other types of articles too such as clinical communication, case reports, technical reports, and letters to editor that the PG students can publish. Nonetheless, the number of manuscripts submitted to indexed journals for publication is increasing day by day. There is a desperate publication race for original articles. In this race of publications, it is likely that one can lose and get frustrated. Nonetheless, one has to be smart to get one's thesis successfully published. Motivation, perseverance, meticulousness, determination, hard and smart work of the student and teacher can be the prime pillars for success in this endeavour.

REFERENCES

1. Dhulkhed VK, Kurdi MS, Dhulkhed PV, Ramaswamy AH. Faculty promotions in medical institutions in India: Can we improve the criteria? Indian J Anaesth. 2016;60(11): 796-800.
2. Bajwa SJ, Sawhney C. Preparing manuscript: Scientific writing for publication. Indian J Anaesth. 2016;60(9):674-8.
3. Kotur PF. How to write a scientific article for a medical journal? Indian J Anaesth. 2002;46:21-5.
4. Kooistra B, Dijkman B, Einhorn TA, Bhandari M. How to design a good case series. J Bone Joint Surg Am. 2009;91(Suppl 3):21-6.
5. Hall GM. Structure of a scientific paper. In: Hall MG (Ed). How to Write a Scientific Paper, 3rd edition. Navarra: BMJ Publishing Group; 2003. pp.1-5.
6. www.ijaweb.org

ANNEXURE 1

Consent form: Part 1

Information for Participants of the Study

Dear Volunteers,

We welcome you and thank you for your keen interest in participation in this research project. Before you participate in this study, it is important for you to understand why this research is being carried out. This form will provide you all the relevant details of this research. It will explain the nature, the purpose, the benefits, the risks, the discomforts, the precautions and the information about how this project will be carried out. It is important that you read and understand the contents of the form carefully. This form may contain certain scientific terms and hence, if you have any doubts or if you want more information, you are free to ask the study personnel or the contact person mentioned below before you give your consent and also at any time during the entire course of the project.

1. Project Title

Effect of low dose tranexamic acid on intraoperative blood loss in neurosurgical patients—a randomised controlled clinical trial.

2. Department and Institute

............XYZ Medical College

3. Name of the Investigator

Dr ABC
PG Junior Resident,
Department of Anaesthesiology, XYZ Medical College

Guide:
Dr DEF
Assistant Professor,
Department of Anaesthesiology, XYZ Medical College

Co-guide:
Dr GHI
Assistant Professor,
Department of Anaesthesiology, XYZ Medical College

4. What is the purpose of this project/study?

To study if low dose tranexamic acid reduces blood loss during surgery and in turn the need for blood transfusion.

5. What is the selection procedure of participants? (Including the inclusion and exclusion criteria)

Inclusion criteria:

- All patients undergoing elective craniotomy of age group 18–60 years
- Belonging to ASA I and II

Exclusion criteria:

- Patients with hepatic or renal disorder
- Patients with bleeding diathesis or abnormal laboratory tests (abnormal PT-INR, platelet count)
- Patient on aspirin a week before surgery
- Patient receiving anticoagulants
- Patients undergoing intracranial vascular surgeries or re-exploratory craniotomy

6. How will it be carried out (procedure of the study)?

You will be assigned to one of the two groups randomly based on computer-generated randomisation chart. You will be explained about the procedure the day before the surgery. About 5–8 mL of blood will be taken from you the day before surgery for some of the lab tests (namely PT-INR, fibrinogen, platelets, electrolytes, and Hb%). If the results come normal you will be taken up for the study. On the day of operation, anaesthesia will be administered using standard protocol and then the drug tranexamic acid will be given intravenously just before the surgery begins and also continued throughout surgery as an infusion.

At the end of operation, the total loss will be estimated. The same laboratory tests will be repeated both during the surgery and immediate postoperatively.

7. What are the responsibilities of participants?

Patients are allowed to decide whether to enter the study or not. After opting in, patients are given full liberty to opt out at any stage. During the study period, participants are expected to extend full cooperation to the investigator.

8. What are the expected risks for the participants?

Tranexamic acid is a very safe drug with very few proven side effects. One of the major complications being thrombosis which is reported to be very rare and almost nil in the dose what we will be using.

9. What are the expected benefits of the research to the participants?

Patients will have significantly less blood loss during the surgery and hence less or no blood transfusion.

10. Will participants be compensated for participation in this trial?

No.

11. Whether my participation in this study be kept confidential?

Yes.

12. Can I withdraw from the study at any time during the study period?

Yes.

13. If there is any new finding/information, would I be informed?
Yes.

14. What happens in case of a study related injury?
In the event of any complication occurring, it will be managed according to the standard practice.

15. Is there any alternative to the treatment mentioned?
Yes. Other drugs such as EACA, aprotinin.

For any study related queries, you are free to contact—

Name of the contact person with official address and phone number:
Dr ABC
Junior Resident,
Department of Anaesthesiology,
XYZ Medical College.
Phone No.: 01234 56789.

Place:

Signature of investigator:

Signature of the participant:

Date:

Witness:

Signature of witness:

Date:

Consent form: Part 2

Participant Consent Form:

Title of the Project: Effect of low dose tranexamic acid on intraoperative blood loss in neurosurgical patients—A randomised controlled clinical trial.

Participant's Name:...

Address: ....
....
....
....

The details of the study have been provided to me, in writing and explained to me by the investigator in my own language. I confirm that I have understood the above study and had the opportunity to ask questions. I understand that my participation in the study is voluntary and that I am free to withdraw at any time without giving any reason, without any medical care or legal rights being affected. I agree not to restrict the use of any data or results that arise from the study provided such a use is only for scientific purpose(s). I have been provided with a copy of the "Consent Form 1 of 2" giving the 'information for participants of the study'. I fully consent to participate in the above study.

Signature of the participant:

.... Date: ....

Signature of the witness:

.... Date: ....

ANNEXURE 2

MASTER CHART - Group M

Date	Name	Age†	Gender	IPN	Procedure	Wgt	Hgt	BMI	MMS	ASA	PR	SBP	DBP	N	Ti
02-11-2022	Prema	40	F	24854	Right PCNL	60	160	23	2	ASA II	88	147	84	1	30
05-11-2022	Geetha	31	F	11356	Right simple mastectomy	60	155	23	2	ASA II	90	150	82	1	30
11-11-2022	Ashok	40	M	11723	Right PCNL	60	160	23.4	2	ASA II	74	143	83	1	25
15-11-2022	Namdev	37	M	22912	L4-L5 laminectomy	80	170	28	2	ASA II	74	150	89	1	25
23-11-2022	Yallappa	44	M	1149	Frey's procedure	55	165	20	2	ASA II	84	142	79	1	30
30-11-2022	Anandiah	36	M	23475	Cystojejunostomy	45	154	19	2	ASA II	89	142	90	1	30
05-12-2022	Mahalingavva	60	F	23650	Left PCNL	42	150	18.6	2	ASA II	93	149	91	1	35
08-12-2022	Jayasheela	60	F	46471	Laparoscopic ovarian cystectomy	60	160	23.4	2	ASA II	73	140	83	1	25
08-12-2022	Girija	43	F	27991	Left modified radical mastectomy	50	156	23.2	2	ASA II	104	144	96	1	25
08-12-2022	Indira	42	F	89830	Right PCNL	70	165	25	2	ASA II	91	143	99	1	20
09-12-2022	Shakuntala	62	F	53733	Left lumpectomy	65	160	25.4	2	ASA II	81	147	91	1	30
10-12-2022	Mahesh	42	M	27109	Lateral pancreaticojejunostomy	55	164	20.4	1	ASA II	101	149	89	1	25
10-12-2022	Md Ali	49	M	55279	Right PCNL	60	165	22.1	2	ASA II	98	149	93	1	25
12-10-2022	Savithri	47	F	53701	Right modified radical mastectomy	56	160	21.8	2	ASA II	100	147	94	1	25
12-12-2022	Farida	41	F	13487	Right modified radical mastectomy	52	153	22.4	1	ASA II	92	144	84	1	30
13-12-2022	Yasmin banu	40	F	13240	Total thyroidectomy	50	150	22.2	2	ASA II	76	136	74	1	30
14-12-2022	Foujiya	45	F	13023	Left modified radical mastectomy	55	156	22.6	2	ASA II	74	144	92	1	25
14-12-2022	Sulochana	59	F	12244	Left modified radical mastectomy	50	150	21.2	2	ASA II	78	144	92	1	25
18-12-2022	Shakira	48	F	10559	Total thyroidectomy	55	152	23.8	2	ASA II	82	139	72	1	30
30-12-2022	Rajiya	42	F	27993	Right pushback PCNL	50	156	21.6	2	ASA II	84	144	87	1	25
05-01-2023	Bhimappa	63	M	28083	Right PCNL	50	158	21.3	2	ASA II	66	142	79	1	25
12-01-2023	Nandeeshwar	37	M	27585	Left PCNL	70	164	24.6	2	ASA II	88	147	89	1	35
15-01-2023	Geetha	55	F	20314	Left PCNL	60	160	23.6	2	ASA II	84	140	90	1	30

†Age in years.

[*Key:* ASA: American Society of Anesthesiologists' class; BMI (kg/sq.m.): body mass index; DBP: diastolic blood pressure (mm Hg); Hgt: height (cm); IPN: in-patient number; MMS: Mallampati score; N: number of attempts; PCNL: percutaneous nephrolithotomy; PR: pulse rate (beats/min); SBP: systolic blood pressure (mm Hg); Ti: time taken for intubation (seconds); Wgt: weight]

ANNEXURE 3

XYZ Medical College, XYZ
Plagiarism Verification Certificate: Part A

1. Name of researcher...
2. Title of thesis...
3. Course...
4. University registration number.........................
5. Name of the guide/supervisor............................
6. Official designation of guide and address..

The above thesis has been scanned for similarity detection. The report is as follows:

Software used:...................................   Date:.........................

Similarity index:.................................   Total word count:................

The report is attached for the review by supervisor.

Signature of Guide/Supervisor

The plagiarism report of the above thesis/dissertation has been reviewed by the undersigned

☐ The similarity is below accepted norms

☐ The similarity is above accepted norms, because of the following reasons:

....

....

Certified that the thesis/dissertation is plagiarism free/the similarity content is within the acceptable limits and does not affect the originality of research work. Therefore, the thesis may be considered for submission to the university. The software report is attached.

Signature of the researcher   Signature of supervisor/guide

XYZ Medical College, XYZ
Plagiarism Verification Certificate: Part B

No. .... Date ....

Certificate

Certified that the thesis entitled...

....

....

of Dr..

Submitted in partial fulfilment of the requirement of postgraduation degree of...................................

Department of...

Has been verified with the Turnitin Similarity Checking Tool of XYZ Medical College, XYZ and found the similarity index is..............................percent.

Supervisor/In Charge

Document Details

Submission ID
trn:oid:::3618:89619854

Submission Date
Apr 4, 2025, 4:50 PM GMT+5:30

Download Date
Apr 4, 2025, 4:52 PM GMT+5:30

File Name
Christa George.docx

File Size
665.3 KB

38 Pages

10,298 Words

61,719 Characters

turnitin Page 1 of 43 - Cover Page Submission ID trn:oid:::3618:89619854

turnitin Page 2 of 43 - Integrity Overview Submission ID trn:oid:::3618:89619854

4% Overall Similarity

The combined total of all matches, including overlapping sources, for each database.

Filtered from the Report

- Bibliography
- Small Matches (less than 14 words)

Match Groups

- 28 Not Cited or Quoted 4%
  Matches with neither in-text citation nor quotation marks
- 0 Missing Quotations 0%
  Matches that are still very similar to source material
- 0 Missing Citation 0%
  Matches that have quotation marks, but no in-text citation
- 0 Cited and Quoted 0%
  Matches with in-text citation present, but no quotation marks

Top Sources

- 3% Internet sources
- 1% Publications
- 1% Submitted works (Student Papers)

Integrity Flags

0 Integrity Flags for Review

No suspicious text manipulations found.

Our system's algorithms look deeply at a document for any inconsistencies that would set it apart from a normal submission. If we notice something strange, we flag it for you to review.

A Flag is not necessarily an indicator of a problem. However, we'd recommend you focus your attention there for further review.

ANNEXURE 4

Study Proforma

Title: Effect of Tranexamic Acid on Intraoperative Blood Loss in Neurosurgical Patients: A randomised Controlled Trial

Name of the patient: ....

Date: ....

Age/Gender: ....

IP No.:

Height (cm): ....

Weight (kg): ....

Diagnosis: ....

Proposed surgery: ....

Study drug: Saline/Tranexamic acid

Starting time: ....

Bolus:

- Starting time: ....
- Ending time: ....

Infusion:

- Starting time: ....
- Ending time: ....

Clinical Parameters Table

Parameters	*Baseline value*	*2 hours*	*4 hours*	*6 hours*	*8 hours*	*10 hours*	*Immediate postoperative*
Heart rate (per min)							
MAP (mm Hg)							
SPO_2 (%)							
Temperature (degree)							
UO (mL)							
Blood loss (mL)							
Blood infused (number of units)							
Crystalloids infused (mL)							
Colloids infused (mL)							

Lab Parameters Table

Parameters	*Baseline value*	*3 hour*	*6 hour*	*9 hour*	*12 hour*	*Immediate postoperative*
Hb %						
PT-INR						
Electrolytes: Na^+						
K^+						
Ca^{++}						
Platelet count (per cu mm)						
Fibrinogen (g/L) (every 4 hours)						
Hct (%)						
POD_5 Hb %						

- Least temperature recorded: .... Its duration: ....
- Minimum MAP recorded: .... Its duration: ....
- Total IV fluids:
    - Crystalloids: ....
    - Colloid: ....
- Total duration of hypotension: ....
- Total blood loss during surgery: ....
- Total blood given: ....
- Other blood products given: ....
- Hb loss = (Hb pre-Hbpost) × BV + Hbt

Intra-/postoperative complications (if any)

1.

2.

3.

(*Note:* Hb: haemoglobin; IV: intravenous; BV: blood volume; PT-INR: prothrombin time-international normalised ratio; UO: urine output; POD: postoperative day; Na^+: sodium; K^+: potassium; Ca^{++}: calcium; Hct: haematocrit; Hbt: amount of haemoglobin that the patient receives through transfusion)

ANNEXURE 5

Example of Ethics Committee Certificate

NATIONAL INSTITUTE OF MENTAL HEALTH AND NEURO SCIENCES
(INSTITUTE OF NATIONAL IMPORTANCE)
P.B. NO. 2900, HOSUR ROAD, BENGALURU - 560 029 (INDIA)

Member-Secretary
NIMHANS ETHICS COMMITTEE

Off: 26995004
Fax: 91-80-26564830/26566811
Email: bng@nimhans.kar.nic.in
kalyanybg@yahoo.com

No. NIMH/DO/ETHICS

'THROUGH HOD AND GUIDE'

1. Name of the investigator:
2. Reference number of the investigator: Letter dated 6/3/15
3. Title of the proposal submitted for ethical clearance:
4. Nature of the proposal submitted for ethical clearance: DM (Neuroanaethesia) Thesis Protocol
5. Date of Ethics Committee meeting held: 23rd March, 2015
6. NIMHANS IEC No. of the proposal: (Please quote this number in all the future correspondence related to this study) Item No. 3.03, Neurosciences
7. Members of the Ethics Sub-Commitee who reviewed the proposal:
8. Clear statement of the decision reached:

Decision: The DM (Neuroanesthesia) Thesis Protocol and study related documents are approved with respect to ethical aspects.

MEMBER – SECRETARY, NIMHANS ETHICS COMMITTEE

ANNEXURE 6

Synopsis Template

Submitted To ....

University ....

Submitted By ....

Under The Guidance Of ....

Proforma for Registration of Subjects for Dissertation		
1.	Name of the candidate and address	
2.	Name of the institution	
3.	Course of study and subject	
4.	Date of admission to the course	
5.	Title of dissertation	
6.	Brief resume of intended work: 6.1 Need for study: 6.2 Review of literature Aim of the study: Objectives of the study: Primary objective: Secondary objectives:	
7.	Materials and methods: 7.1 Source of data: 7.2 Methods of data collection: Study design: Study period: Sample Sample size: Formula used for sample size calculation: Inclusion criteria: Exclusion criteria:	

	Method of study: Statistical analysis: 7.3 Does the study require any investigation or intervention to be conducted on patients or animals specific? 7.4 Has the ethical clearance been obtained from ethical committee of your institution in case of 7.3?	
8.	References: (In the style specified by the University)	
9.	Signature of candidate	
10.	Remarks of the guide	
11.	11.1 Name and designation of the guide	
	11.2 Signature of guide	
	11.3 Head of the Department	
	11.4 Signature of Head of Department	
12.	12.1 Remarks of Chairman and Principal	Name, address and mail id of the Principal Remarks:
	12.2 Signature of Principal	

ANNEXURE 7

Example of a Search Strategy for Review of Literature

A. Keywords:
   1. Palm print sign
   2. Difficult airway
   3. Diabetes mellitus
   4. Limited joint mobility (LJM)
   5. Airway assessment tools
   6. Airway indices
   7. Mallampati test
   8. Thyromental distance (TMD)
   9. Upper lip bite test (ULBT)

B. Medical Subject Headings (MeSH) Terms:
   1. 'Palm Print Sign'
   2. 'Diabetes Mellitus'
   3. 'Difficult Airway'
   4. 'Airway Management'
   5. 'Joint Mobility'
   6. 'Mallampati Score'
   7. 'Thyromental Distance'
   8. 'Airway Obstruction'

C. Filters:
   1. Language: English
   2. Population: Human Studies
   3. Age group: Adults (18–65 years)
   4. Study design:
      - Case-control studies
      - Cohort studies
      - Observational studies
      - Retrospective studies
   5. Publication type:
      - Full-text articles
      - Peer-reviewed journals
   6. Publication date: Last 10 years (2013–2023)

D. Databases to search:
   1. PubMed
   2. Scopus
   3. Web of Science
   4. Cochrane Library
   5. Google Scholar

E. Boolean search strings (examples):
   1. 'Palm print sign' and 'difficult airway' and 'diabetes mellitus'
   2. ('Palm print sign' or 'limited joint mobility') and 'airway assessment tools' and 'diabetes'
   3. ('Airway indices' and 'Mallampati test') and ('difficult intubation' or 'airway obstruction')
   4. 'Thyromental distance' and 'upper lip bite test' and 'diabetes mellitus'
   5. ('Airway management' and 'diabetes mellitus') and ('palm print sign' or 'airway management')

F. Exclusion criteria in search:
   1. Studies on paediatric populations
   2. Animal studies
   3. Article published in non-peer reviewed journals
   4. Case reports without original data
   5. Non-English publications

Note: The study topic is related to the palm print sign in the preoperative assessment of difficult airway in patients with diabetes mellitus.

ANNEXURE 8

Copyright Declaration by the Candidate

I hereby declare that the XYZ Medical College, XYZ shall have the right to preserve, use and disseminate the dissertation/thesis in print or electronic format for academic/research purposes.

Place: XYZ

Date:

Signature:

Dr
PG Trainee in Anaesthesiology
XYZ Medical College, XYZ

ANNEXURE 9

Sample Abstract of a Scientific Paper

Clinically Alarming Reflex Bradycardia during Lumbar Spine Surgery: A Retrospective Observational Study

Background and Objectives

Haemodynamic perturbations which include severe bradycardia following lumbar spine surgery are not common.[1] They usually occur intraoperatively when the patient is positioned prone for surgery. If left unattended, they can lead to transient cardiovascular episodes which may further progress, resulting in dreadful outcomes.[2,3]

The objective of our study was to find out the incidence of such cardiovascular episodes and the probable reason in patients undergoing lumbar spine surgery.

Methods

This retrospective observational study analysed medical records of 142 patients who underwent lumbar decompressive surgery for degenerative changes and disc herniation between January 2022 and August 2023. Other cases such as lumbar spine surgeries for tumours and trauma were excluded.

Results

Bradycardia (lowest 28 beats/min) was observed intraoperatively in 22 patients (15 male and 7 female) aged between 16 and 75 years. The occurrence of clinically significant bradycardia was seen in 15.50% (22/142) of patients undergoing lumbar spine surgery when handling of stretched and compromised nerve root was done by the surgical team.

As soon as the surgical stimulus was removed and the stretched nerve route handling was stopped, bradycardia improved, and heart rate became normal in 13.38% (19/142) patients. However, 2.12% (3/142) patients needed treatment with anticholinergic drugs. All the patients had successful recovery without any postoperative neurological deficit.

Conclusion

Awareness of such incidents in the surgical team can help to prevent catastrophic outcomes caused by adverse cardiac events. Further research is needed to evaluate the exact aetiology which can lead to haemodynamic changes in lumbar spine surgery.

References

1. Weimer JM, Marinov M, Avitsian R. Dural traction is a possible cause of hemodynamic changes during single-level transforaminal lumbar interbody fusion. World Neurosurg. 2017;97:761.e1-761.e3.
2. Chowdhury T, Petropolis A, Cappellani RB. Cardiac emergencies in neurosurgical patients. Biomed Res Int. 2015;2015:751320.
3. Chowdhury T, Schaller B. The negative chronotropic effect during lumbar spine surgery: a systemic review and aggregation of an emerging model of spinal cardiac reflex. Medicine (Baltimore). 2017;96(1):e5436.

ANNEXURE 10

Sample Poster

LABOUR ANALGESIA IN PULMONARY HYPERTENSION DUE TO LEFT PULMONARY ARTERY STENOSIS: A BOON WHERE ANAESTHESIA IS A BANE.

SDM

Truth Liberates

AUTHOR: DR. MILON V. MITRAGOTRI (ASSISTANT PROFESSOR) DR. RAVI BHAT (ASSOCIATE PROFESSOR)

DEPARTMENT OF ANAESTHESIA AND PAIN MEDICINE.

INSTITUTE AND POSTAL ADDRESS: SDM MEDICAL COLLEGE AND HOSPITAL, MANJUSHRI NAGAR, SATTUR, DHARWAR.

INTRODUCTION:

- Labour analgesia by epidural route - safe, versatile and painless vaginal delivery in complicated obstetric cases.
- 22year old primigravida with 39 weeks gestation with breech presentation with recently diagnosed untreated severe pulmonary hypertension posted for emergency caesarean section.

We report the successful management of the same using combined spinal epidural labour analgesia with good maternal and fetal outcomes.

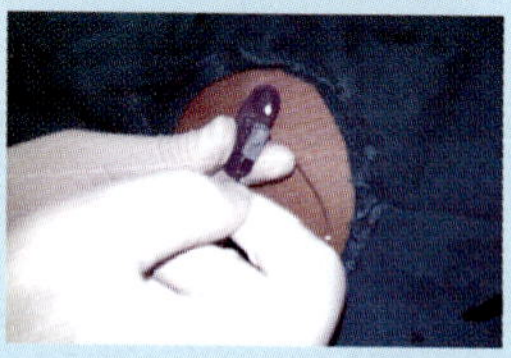

CASE REPORT.

Clincal History

- Frequent syncopal attacks, chest pain, NYHA III dyspnoea and diaphoresis since childhood.
- No history of paroxysmal nocturnal dyspnoea or pedal edema.

Physical Examination

- PR-80/min, BP- 138/72mmHg, SpO_2 of 90% on room air, Respiratory rate of 32/min.
- Pansystolic murmur in the mitral area and an ejection systolic murmur in the pulmonary area (Grade-3)
- RS- bilateral occasional basal crepitations with equal vesicular breath sounds in both lung fields.

INVESTIGATIONS

- ECG revealed right axis deviation with prominent R wave in aVR.
- 2D-ECHO done prior to conception at a clinic outside revealed pulmonary valve doming, severe valvular left pulmonary artery stenosis, transpulmonary gradient **138mmHg!!!**
- Recent 2D-ECHO done 3 months also revealed a mild mitral valve prolapse with normal

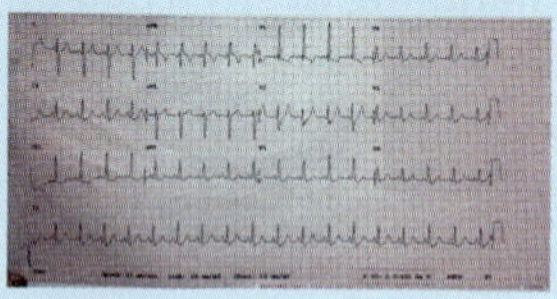

PROCEDURE

- Irrespective of the fetal outcome, written informed consent was taken for vaginal delivery under labour epidural analgesia.
- Pulse oximetry, ECG and NIBP, 18G cannula in situ. Simple face mask with 2L/min.
- Combined spinal (25ug fentanyl) followed by epidural analgesia
- Epidural catheter of 20G inserted after confirmation by loss of resistance and fixed at 9cm
- No test dose was given.
- 0.1% bupivacaine 8cc bolus was given followed by an infusion of the 0.1%bupivacaine with fentanyl(2ug/ml) at the rate of 4ml/hr.
- Systemic hemodynamics, pain relief and fetal heart rate monitored.
- Phenylephrine -treat any episode of hypotension.
- Oxygen saturation was maintained above 95%.
- No hypotension or fetal bradycardia noted.
- LBW male child 1.9kg was delivered by assisted forceps extraction 4 hours later with an APGAR score of 5 and 9 at 1 & 5 mins respectively. Baby shifted to NICU for three days for observation for transient tachpnoea and healthy mother and baby were discharged 4days later.
- Patient was advised against conception again albeit a cardiac surgery is done.

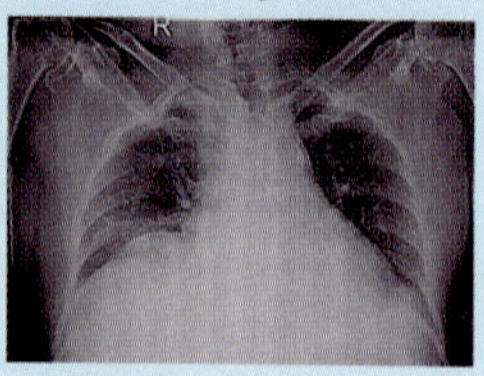

DISCUSSION

- Pulmonary Hypertension is **defined** as a mean pulmonary artery pressure (PAP) >25mmHg at rest with a pulmonary capillary wedge pressure<12mmHg.
- **Predictors for poor prognosis** in PAH include poor functional status, poor exercise capacity, elevated right atrial pressure, significant right ventricular (RV)dysfunction, RV failure, low cardiac index, elevated brain natriuretic peptide(BNP).[1] PAH due to congenital heart disease have a relatively better prognosis. The transpulmonary valve gradient due to left pulmonary valve stenosis in our case was **138mmHg** which was quite high. Our search did not yield any previous case reports of such high gradient.
- Surgery for patients with pulmonary hypertension is associated with significant morbidity and mortality regardless of the anaesthetic technique utilized.
- **Management** of the patient with pulmonary hypertension begins with treatment of the underlying cause and symptomatic therapy, including diuretics for volume overload and oxygen to maintain arterial saturation above 90%[1] Percutaneous pulmonary valve implantation may be an option for patients with severe pulmonary regurgitation and pulmonary hypertension associated with congenital heart disease.[4]
- Pregnancy in women with pulmonary hypertension stresses the already compromised cardiovascular system.
- Harsoor et al report successful management of a patient with pulmonary hypertension under epidural anaesthesia[2]
- Suresh B et al reported successful maternal and fetal outcomes with segmental epidural analgesia in a patient with ventricular septal outcome with pulmonary hypertension.[3]

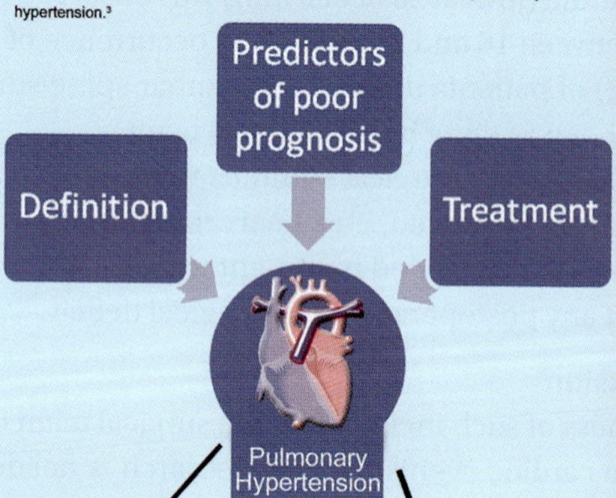

Advantages of labour analgesia
- Greater versatility of effect
Reduces Maternal cartecholamine levels
-Stress of labour minimised
-Decreased PVR
-Decreased adrenergic stimulation
-Increased uteroplacental circulation

Goals of labour analgesia
to maintain adequate preload, systemic vascular resistance (SVR) and contractility in order to allow the right ventricle to maintain cardiac output

to prevent increases in PVR from hypoxia, hypercarbia, acidosis, agitation, pain and hypothermia.

CONCLUSION:

Labour analgesia by epidural route can be a boon in pregnancy complicated with pulmonary hypertension where surgery under anaesthesia is befit with morbidity and mortality. Under adequate preparation and precautions with assistance of obstetricians, labour analgesia can save the day by maintaning stable systemic hemodynamics.

REFERENCES

1. Chad D. Pritts, Ronald G. P. Anaesthesia for patients with pulmonary hypertension. Current Opinion in Anaesthesiology 2010, 23:411-416.
2. Anaesthetic management of parturient with pulmonary hypertension posted for caserean section- a case report. Dr. Harsoor S.S., Dr. Joshi Suyajna D. Indian J. Anaesth. 2005 : 223-225.
3. Suresh B. Mridula P. Epidural analgesia in the intrapartum management of a patient with ventricular septal defect with pulmonary hypertension-a case report. Indian J. Anaesth. 2002; 46(5) 405-408.

ANNEXURE 11

Postgraduate Examiner's Report of the Dissertation

XYZ Medical College, XYZ Place

(To be detached and returned to this office)
E-mail: xyz@gmail.com

Name of the candidate: ....

Subject: ....

College: ....

Title of the Dissertation: ....

Report of the Examiner: March/April, 2025

1. General Observations on the Dissertation:
2. Please state whether the Dissertation is approved or not approved by you (kindly tick the appropriate box):

   [ ] Approved

   [ ] Not Approved
3. If not approved, please suggest the lines on which the Dissertation has to be revised before resubmission:

Date: ....

Name, Address of the Examiner: ....

Signature of the Examiner: ....

Frequently Asked Questions Regarding Dissertation

Maneesha Godbole, Madhuri S Kurdi

FREQUENTLY ASKED QUESTIONS BY A POSTGRADUATE STUDENT REGARDING A DISSERTATION

1. **What is the aim of doing a dissertation?**
   Dissertation shows the ability of a student to perform research. This is one of the criteria to become eligible to obtain a postgraduate degree.
2. **What is a synopsis?**
   Synopsis is an overview of the research that a student plans to undertake.
3. **How should I find a good topic for my dissertation?**
   A good topic can come from questions asked about the health and illness that one observes in the community or clinical setting. What, why, when, where, who, and how are the questions that can give a good topic. For example: How can health workers diagnose malnutrition in the field? This gave us the 'road to health' card with the coloured bands.

   Another way to get a good topic is by browsing journals of the relevant speciality.

   One can also consult the guide who may suggest a good topic.
4. **What are the common reasons for rejection of synopsis by the university?**
   The common reasons are—incomplete title, poorly framed objectives, incorrect sample size, and inappropriate statistical tests.
5. **Can I calculate sample size myself or should I go to a statistician?**
   It is better to take the help of the statistician. Calculate by yourself first and then go to the statistician. This will help you learn better by identifying the mistakes in your calculation.
6. **Is it mandatory to register every study thesis in the Clinical Trials Registry of India (CTRI)?**
   A study that requires intervention needs to be registered.
7. **When should I start recruiting the study subjects?**
   It is better to start recruiting subjects after the synopsis has been accepted by the university and CTRI registration is done.
8. **What is the difference between Bibliography and References?**
   Bibliography is a list of all the sources that one has looked up (consulted), with regard to the study.

   References is a list of all sources from which one has quoted a fact (cited) in writing up the dissertation.
9. **How should I procure latest scientific references related to my dissertation?**
   Scientific and valid online search engines should be used to browse the available literature. Unpublished material available in the department or library, such as students projects or postgraduate dissertation, should also be referred.

10. **How should I keep in touch with my guide during the study period?**
You should consult and keep the guide informed at every step of the study. A guide is usually physically present in the department. In case you are not able to meet up with the guide, you should keep connected through phone or email.

11. **What should I do if my synopsis gets rejected?**
Whenever a synopsis is rejected, the reasons are listed. Modify the synopsis to rectify the mistakes and resubmit.

12. **What should I do if my dissertation gets rejected?**
If one has been thorough and honest in carrying out the study, rarely is a dissertation rejected. Being fully prepared and well versed with your study will help you to defend your findings. However, if you are not able to defend your results, you should accept the rejection, find out what mistakes you have made and resubmit it. The examiner will usually mention the reasons for rejecting the dissertation.

13. **What should I do if the study of my dissertation yields negative results?**
It is a misconception that a study is good only if it gives a positive result. Accepting a null hypothesis to disprove assumptions is equally important in enriching the medical knowledge.

14. **What should I do if my guide is impatient with me?**
One should always be fully oriented to what is being done, never go unprepared, and have immense patience and persistence. There has to be a reason if the guide is impatient with you. Try to identify and rectify this.

15. **Should I present the study of my dissertation as a paper in a conference or should I send it for publication in a journal? When can I publish my dissertation in a scientific journal?**
You can present the dissertation study as a paper/poster first in a state/national conference. You can submit it to a scientific journal for publication after your dissertation is accepted by your university. You should mention during submission to the journal that this was a postgraduate dissertation. Consult your postgraduate guide and choose the journal that you are going to submit your study. Your guide can help you in writing the manuscript. Do not ever forget to put your postgraduate guide's name as an author. The order of the authors is left to yourself and your guide.

FREQUENTLY ASKED QUESTIONS BY A POSTGRADUATE GUIDE REGARDING A DISSERTATION

1. **What exactly does 'guiding' the student for a dissertation mean?**
'Guiding' means supporting, giving ideas, correcting the mistakes, motivating and teaching at various steps of the preparation of the dissertation. Your role starts with finding and approving the topic of the dissertation and ends with your approval of the written dissertation (when you sign on the certificate of completion of the dissertation which states that the dissertation was written under your supervision and guidance). You need to help the student write the synopsis, defend the student and the study in case controversies/ queries are raised by the ethics committee, help the student to revise and resubmit the synopsis in case of rejection, guide the preparation of the study protocol, supervise the recruitment of cases for the study, supervise the collection of data and help in application of appropriate statistical tests.

You finally need to go through what the student has written under various subheadings of the dissertation and ensure that there are no language errors, no plagiarism and the review of literature is complete with all latest references. You need to meticulously go through the master chart, observations and results obtained after the application of statistical tests. Students need expert guidance for writing the 'Discussion' part.

2. **How should I find a good/suitable dissertation topic for my student?**
   Keep a diary in which you can keep on jotting down research ideas that come to you. This will help you to find the topic when the student is allotted to you. Keep reading articles that are published from time to time in the journals of your speciality. Sometimes, review articles on a topic can give you novel ideas for research. Attending conferences regularly to understand the current issues can help to comprehend the current state of evidence. Plan a novel study that is feasible in your setup. Do not plan a 'me too study', wherein one just changes some drug doses or adds another study group to an already published study. Topics of dissertations already submitted to various universities/colleges are available on the university/college websites.
3. **What should I do if the student appears disinterested/is insincere in collecting data?**
   Explain politely to the student the value of collecting data sincerely. Tell him/her that many scientific journals will ask for the production of raw data. It is easy for journal editors to detect manipulated data. The conclusion drawn from studies with manipulated data is not valid and can be dangerous if applied in clinical practice. Tell the student that the dissertation is prepared usually once in a person's lifetime. Hence, one needs to be sincere while working on it.
4. **Should the student write all headings of the dissertation after completion of the study or in between?**
   The Title, Aims, and Objectives are ready when the synopsis is prepared. The Review of Literature can be written in the first few months. The student can keep searching for latest information published on this topic and keep adding this to the Review of Literature. Once the data collection is complete and the results of the application of statistical results are available, the Discussion and Conclusion parts can be written.
5. **How can one look for plagiarism in the dissertation? How much of plagiarism is acceptable?**
   A maximum of 10% similarity is acceptable. One can use Plagiarism Detection Tools such as iThenticate, Turnitin, and Plagiarism.org. Universities may specify which plagiarism detection tool is to be used.
6. **What is the maximum and minimum number of pages permissible in a dissertation?**
   There is no universal rule for this as such. The length of the dissertation depends on the topic, the number of references related to the topic, the depth of review of literature and the number of observations and groups in the study. Usually, a dissertation contains 100–200 pages.
7. **What is the minimum/maximum number of references permissible for the Bibliography section? How recent should be the references?**
   There is no universal rule for this as such. The number of references depends on the novelty of the topic, the field of the study

and the depth of the student's research. It can vary from 50 to 200. Each university may have specific rules regarding the number of references.

8. **Can a topic of the dissertation which is already conducted in a department/ university be repeated? If so, after how many years?**
The topic and methodology should not be exactly the same as previously done by another student. Your research should have something novel, such as new methodology with novel equipment/technology, different data collection methods and analytical techniques or a different study population/ geographical area. The rules and policies regarding repetition of the topic vary from university to university.

9. **Can a student make use of artificial intelligence (AI) in research and dissertation writing?**
Yes. AI can be used as a tool for assistance. You can generate research ideas by using the AI tool as a brainstorming partner and prompt the AI with ideas and vice versa. Large language models can give an overview of existing literature that is freely available on a topic. You can search research databases using AI platforms. Generative AI and Large Language Models, like ChatGPT®, Microsoft Co-Pilot®, and Google Gemini® are available. AI technology can be utilised for language editing, grammar check and statistical analysis.

It is, however, important that the use of AI is done in a responsible manner. AI generated responses may include passages verbatim from other sources amounting to plagiarism. Generative AI may not always produce accurate results and may sometimes create false new data. One should not upload sensitive research data to an open AI platform because it can become a part of that model's data and be later used by the model to provide responses to another person's queries regarding the topic. Use of AI manipulated scientific images can amount to research misconduct.

Universities and scientific journals nowadays make it mandatory for the student/author to make a written disclosure regarding the use of AI technology that was used in the conduct of the study and writing of the thesis/manuscript.

10. **How can one find out if AI models have been used for text generation?**
AI Text Classifier, GPTzero can be used.

11. **Which software can be used for randomisation, data collection, data storage and statistical analysis?**
For randomisation, one can use OpenEPI software.

For data collection and storage, one can use Epicollect5 software.

Epi Info is a free public software developed by Centers for Disease Control and Prevention (CDC), USA that researchers can use to collect, analyse and report data apart from designing a questionnaire, managing data entries, performing statistical analysis and providing graphs. Software such as Statistical Package for the Social Sciences (SPSS) (paid) and JAMOVI (free) can be used only for analysis. JAMOVI is suitable for both beginners and advanced researchers. It supports a wide range of statistical tests including descriptive statistics (means, medians, standard deviations and distributions), inferential statistics (t-tests, ANOVA, Chi-square tests), regression (linear, logistic and mixed models) and advanced models. SPSS can be used to import and clean large datasets, perform descriptive statistics (mean, median, standard deviation, frequency distribution), inferential statistical tests (t-tests, Chi-square tests, ANOVA) and to generate charts and graphs.

12. **What is the difference between a 'trial' and a 'study'?**
'Trials' are specific types of experimental studies which involve a newer treatment (testing a new drug/studying a new surgical technique) or active intervention. 'Study' is a general term for any investigation to answer a research question. It can include observational studies, case studies, epidemiological studies, etc. All trials are studies, but all studies are not trials.

13. **Can postgraduate students conduct research studies other than the one of their dissertation?**
Yes. The students can do it. They can plan the study, present the synopsis before the institutional ethics committee, get the study registered in the clinical trials registry and go ahead.

Index

Page numbers followed by *b* refer to box, *f* refer to figure, *fc* refer to flowchart, and *t* refer to table.

I

K

L

M

N

O

P